Ethics Committees: A Challenge for Catholic Health Care

Contributors

The following persons participated in the September 8-9, 1983 workshop. The authors' contributions appear in Part 2 and the panelists' in Part 3.

Authors: Paul W. Armstrong, JD, LLM
Counsellor at Law for the Karen Quinlan Family
Morristown, NJ

Rev. Benedict Ashley, OP, PhD, STM
Professor of Moral Theology, Acquinas Institute
St. Louis, MO

Sr. Miriam Therese Larkin, CSJ, PhD
General Superior, Sisters of St. Joseph of Carondelet
St. Louis, MO

Most Rev. Daniel E. Pilarczyk, PhD, STD, DD
Archbishop of Cincinnati
Cincinnati, OH

Sr. Mary Roch Rocklage, RSM
Provincial Administrator, Sisters of Mercy of the Union
St. Louis, MO

Panelists:

Frank J. Brescia, MD
Calvary Hospital
New York, NY

Rev. Robert E. Lampert
Oblate School of Theology
San Antonio, TX

Martha Lehmann, RN
St. Joseph's Hospital
St. Paul, MN

Rev. Joseph T. Mangan, SJ
Holy Cross Hospital
Chicago, IL

Rev. Thomas J. O'Donnell, SJ
St. Francis Hospital
Tulsa, OK

Rev. Ted C. W. Smits
Alberta Diocesan
   Medical-Moral Committee
Calgary, Alberta, Canada

Sr. Mary Ellen Vaughn, CSC, RN
Holy Cross Health System
South Bend, IN

Ethics Committees: A Challenge for Catholic Health Care

Edited by
Sister Margaret John Kelly, DC, PhD
Vice President, Mission Services
The Catholic Health Association

and
The Reverend Donald G. McCarthy, PhD
Director of Education
The Pope John XXIII Medical-Moral Research
and Education Center

The Pope John XXIII Medical-Moral Research and Education Center
St. Louis, MO
and
The Catholic Health Association of the United States
St. Louis, MO

Nihil Obstat
  Robert F. Coerver

Imprimatur
  E. J. O'Donnell
  Auxiliary Bishop of St. Louis
  May 1, 1984

Copyright 1984
by
The Catholic Health Association of the United States
St. Louis, MO 63134
and
The Pope John XXIII Medical-Moral Research and Education Center
St. Louis, MO 63134

Library of Congress Cataloging in Publication Data
Main entry under title:

Ethics committees.

  Bibliography: p.
  1. Medical ethics—Congresses. 2. Ethics
committees—Congresses. 3. Medicine—Religious
aspects—Catholic Church—Congresses.
I. Kelly, Margaret John. II. McCarthy, Donald G. III. Catholic
Health Association of the United States. IV. Pope
John XXIII Medical-Moral Research and Education
Center.
R724.E8214   1984   174'.2   84-9635
ISBN 0-87125-096-9

Contents

Preface

Although the application of ethics to medical practice is as old as the Hippocratic oath, recent events have heightened general awareness of the ethical challenges, and even dilemmas, inherent in contemporary medical practice. The technological imperative, "if we are able to do it, we must do it," is being questioned as to its efficacy, and high cost/high technology care is being questioned as to its long-term economy. The disproportionate consumption of resources by the rapidly expanding aged population is also raising questions on the appropriate allocation of limited resources. Media coverage of the celebrated Karen Quinlan, Infant-Baby Doe, and Elizabeth Bouvia cases has removed ethical discussions from the intimate patient-family-physician triad and placed them squarely in the public forum. A recent federal proposal that special review boards be established to monitor the care of infants stimulated great industry controversy, many columns of editorials, and a flood of letters and phone calls supporting both sides of the issue. Thus, the ethical thread running through the efficacy, economy, and efficiency issues is becoming more conspicuous to both professionals and the public.

In such an environment, even facilities with well-articulated and longstanding ethical traditions recognize the need to anticipate difficult ethical situations so that serious, responsible reflection will precede critical decision-making experiences. Over the past two years, the staff of The Catholic Health Association, Division of Mission Services, and The Pope John XXIII Medical-Moral Research and Education Center have collaborated on several projects to assist their members to address these issues. This publication reflects their consulting, research, and educational activities in one area of response--the ethics committee at the institutional, diocesan, and multi-institutional system levels. Ethics committees, whose role is sometimes referred to as "preventive ethics," can assist individuals and institutions in educating to and developing the appropriate policies and protocols to deal with these increasingly complex situations.

This volume, although incorporating some related materials, concentrates heavily on the presentations and experiences of a workshop conducted by CHA and PJC on September 8 and 9, 1983, entitled "The Role and Formation of Ethics Committees in Catholic Health Care." The workshop examined both the theory and practice of developing and implementing ethics committees at the institutional, diocesan, and system levels. Sr. Joan Kalchbrenner, RHSJ, an intern in ethics within the CHA Division of Mission Services during the summer of 1983, contributed significantly to the development of materials for the workshop and this publication.

Part I, "Contemporary Challenges: Ethical Concerns in Health Care," traces the historical development of Catholic medical ethics and describes the current status of ethics committees within CHA member hospitals and at the national level.

Part II, "Contemporary Context: Issues Facing Ethics Committees," provides the theoretical basis for ethics committees presented by five speakers at the workshop on Sept. 8, 1983. The Most Reverend Daniel E. Pilarczyk, PhD, STD, DD, archbishop of Cincinnati, speaks of the Church as teacher and the role of the diocesan bishop in applying the *Ethical and Religious Directives for Catholic Health Facilities* of the National Conference of Catholic Bishops. Rev. Benedict Ashley, OP, a professor of moral theology at the Aquinas Institute of St. Louis, presents an analysis of ethical methodology as used in the application of Catholic teaching to medical-moral issues and critiques the proportionalist approach. Mr. Paul Armstrong, JD, attorney for Karen Quinlan, surveys legislative and judicial trends that foster or affect the formation of ethics committees. Sr. Miriam Therese Larkin, CSJ, Superior General of the Sisters of St. Joseph of Carondelet, and Sr. Mary Roch Rocklage, RSM, Provincial of the Sisters of Mercy of St. Louis, examine the way health care sponsors and institutions develop a corporate conscience and encourage its incorporation into the work of ethics committees.

Part III of this book, "Contemporary Response: Formation and Function of Ethics Committees," summarizes the actual discussion of the formation and functions of ethics committees as presented in the workshop on Sept. 9, 1983. The many practical suggestions presented by the participants, as well as basic legal and philosophical principles, are incorporated into this chapter, which concludes with the presentation of a model institutional committee developed out of participants' observations and presentations and a summary of the advantages and disadvantages of the various models. This model can be adapted for acute and long-term care facilities.

Part IV, "References and Resources," provides materials for both the development and evaluation of ethics committees. In addition to presenting several models of committees and job descriptions of ethicists at the institutional, diocesan, and system levels, the final section includes a glossary of terms for committees and a bibliography of articles on the subject.

At the conclusion of each of the presentations in Part II and at the end of Part III, the issues, questions, and observations raised by participants at the workshop are presented so that readers will gain insights into the broad range of concerns articulated.

Although the future of ethics committees as a means to meet the increasing challenge of providing truly humane and Christian health care cannot be clearly foreseen, this volume may serve as a guidebook along that path as institutions, dioceses, and health care systems develop and evaluate their own responses to contemporary ethical concerns in Catholic health care.

Part One
Contemporary Challenge: Ethical Concerns in Catholic Health Care

Introduction

Ethical concerns have characterized Catholic health care from its beginnings. One Biblical characteristic for identifying worthiness for the kingdom of heaven included neighbor love in caring for the sick: "I was ill and you comforted me" (Mt 25:36). That ethical principle of neighbor love, rather than any vision of power, profit, or prestige, called into existence the Catholic health care apostolate.

The commitment to Catholic ethics that permeates Catholic health care facilities promotes a countercultural posture in the face of increasing secular tendencies to subordinate ethics to law and to identify morality with legality. The effort to separate Church and state unfortunately leads some thinkers to assume that ethics, considered only as a matter of religious preference or private conviction, must be ignored by law and public policy in a pluralistic democracy. Public schools are being told to teach *about* ethics rather than to teach ethics.

Catholic teaching, on the other hand, insists that philosophical ethics, as a study of right and wrong in human behavior based on common human experience, precedes law and envisions the good society that law and public policy seek to realize.

Biblical revelation and Catholic teaching clarify philosophical ethics by tracing the origins of human goodness to the good God and by showing how Christ overcame sin to restore grace and goodness. Evil and injustice can be recognized even in philosophical ethics, but without the clarity and comprehension of religious and Christian ethics. Hence the current U.S. trend to isolate law and public policy from both religious and philosophical ethics cannot advance the good of society nor the good of health care institutions dedicated to the good of the individual.

Catholic health care institutions in the United States, of course, have the freedom to establish their own policies in full accord with philosophical ethics as transformed and clarified by faith and Church teaching. Court decisions such as *Doe v. Bridgeton Hospital Association* have recognized that a privately operated health care facility may follow the ethical norms adopted in its charter and bylaws.[1]

Furthermore, Catholic medical-moral teaching has had an impressive historic importance within Catholic health care facilities and has been included in their charters and bylaws.

The Development of Catholic Medical Ethics

Four specific phases mark the development of Catholic medical ethics within Catholic health care facilities in the United States.[2]

1. Since the seventeenth century, medical ethics has been a recognized division of Catholic moral theology. A well-developed body of medical-moral teaching emerged within the Church, using its natural moral law heritage in a more detailed and systematic way than in other traditions of Christian, religious, or secular ethics. This teaching recognized patients' and health care professionals' moral rights and responsibilities, the justification of surgery and experimentation for the patient's therapeutic benefit, and exceptionless moral norms forbidding mercy killing and direct abortion.

2. The Church's magisterium has taught this theological medical-moral doctrine in an authoritative manner. Pope Pius XII addressed countless medical-moral issues during his papacy (1939 to 1958), and Pope John Paul II has frequently reaffirmed Catholic teaching on the sacredness of human life and its implications. In recent years, the Sacred Congregation for the Doctrine of the Faith has published detailed documents on abortion (1974), sexual ethics (1975), and euthanasia (1980) as well as an explicit reply to questions of the National Conference of Catholic Bishops (NCCB) on sterilization (1975). *The Ethical and Religious Directives for Catholic Health Facilities* (NCCB, 1971) provided 33 specific ethical norms and 10 specific directives for Catholic health care facilities. In their pastoral "Health and Health Care" (NCCB, 1981), the bishops identified and stressed the moral responsibility of each individual to adopt a healthy life style.

3. Catholic health care facilities have recognized their responsibility to develop an "institutional conscience." They have claimed their First Amendment right to uphold religious and ethical principles in their health care service (e.g., in not providing abortion or sterilization services). They have also

sought to assist patients to make informed health care decisions, especially about using ethically extraordinary means of prolonging life. They have recognized their legal and moral liability for their medical services and their obligation to foster communication with family members, who in an ethical sense are patients' proxy representatives. Chaplaincy and pastoral care services have focused on the family as the unit of care.

4. The *Evaluative Criteria for Catholic Health Care Facilities* (The Catholic Health Association, 1980) has stressed medical-moral guidance and education and social justice education as essential to Catholic identity (principles 5 to 7). The criteria for patient care and pastoral care stress the wholistic approach to treatment and an interdisciplinary coordination of institutional services for the patient's total good (principles 3 and 4). The criterion for Christian management has stressed reverence for life and Christian stewardship, basic considerations in the ethics of resource allocation (principle 2).

The Development of Medical-Moral Committees

In the light of deep-rooted ethical concerns and the richness of the Catholic medical-moral heritage, Catholic health care facilities have not hesitated to focus institutional attention on ethical issues. The formulation of the *Ethical and Religious Directives for Catholic Health Facilities* by the NCCB in 1971 was preceded by the earlier versions of that medical-moral charter, especially the *Code of Medical Ethics for Catholic Hospitals* of 1954.

The implementation of such directives could not be automatically ensured even when individual institutions adopted them in charter and bylaws; however, conscientious administrators, who, until the last decade, were usually members of the sponsoring religious communities, made serious efforts to conform institutional policies and practices to these directives. In recent years increasing numbers of laypeople have entered leadership roles in Catholic health care facilities, the number of physicians not of the Catholic faith has increased greatly, and the number of nurses trained in Catholic diploma schools has decreased greatly. New and complex ethical issues have emerged because of advancing medical and scientific achievements. All these factors have stimulated interest in forming or revitalizing medical-moral committees.

CHA's 1981 annual survey (1980 data), completed by almost all CHA member hospitals, included questions on each facility's use of ethicists and moral theologians.[3] The 1983 annual survey (1982 data) included questions on the existence, function, and chairpersons of ethics committees as well as on the use of ethicists and moral theologians and the relationship of institutional committees to the diocese.

The 1983 survey revealed that 228, or 41 percent, of the responding institutions or 36 percent of all Catholic hospitals (559 respondents out of a universe of 630 Catholic hospitals) had ethics committees in 1982; 32 percent of the responding hospitals had an ethicist or a moral theologian available to them, either full or part time during 1982. While at this writing returns of the 1984 CHA survey (1983 data) are not complete, it is interesting to note that approximately 50 percent of the respondent institutions (247 out of 490) reported having ethics committees in place. It is significant that the number of institutions with ethicists or moral theologians increased from 12 percent in the 1981 survey to 32 percent in the 1983 survey but that the number of full-time ethicists had dramatically decreased. It is also important to note that 16 percent of the reporting institutions had both committees and ethicists and that 7 percent had an ethicist without a committee. The questionnaires also revealed that ethics (medical-moral) committees and expertise exist at the corporate and diocesan levels and relate to the individual institutions.

The chart below indicates, according to bed size, the percentage of Catholic hospitals with medical-moral committees as of 1983:

Number of Beds	Percentage with Medical-moral Committees
0-99	22
100-249	37
250-349	45
350-449	47
450-549	67
550 +	50

The particular structure of each facility's medical-moral committee varies according to local circumstances. Some committees are board committees, other are established within the administration or the medical staff, and others draw their members from various disciplines. If the committee is interdisciplinary, it may include only staff members of the institutions or it may also include other members from outside the facility.

The 1982 data gathered in the CHA survey indicated the various functions of these existing committees by percentage:

Policy making	17
Decision making	19
Educational programming	56
Policy recommending	79
Advisory	84

This review of the current functioning of ethics committees in Catholic health care facilities demonstrates the high level of interest these institutions have in the ethical aspects of health care. It suggests that Catholic facilities have pioneered in this area. Recently the President's Commission for the Study of Ethical Problems in Medicine and Biomedical and Behavioral Research commissioned a national survey of hospital ethics committees.[4] That survey extrapolated from its surveys of 602 sample hospitals and concluded that "approximately 1 percent of all hospitals in the United States have ethics committees.[5] It described an ethics committee as one "involved in the decision-making process in specific cases." In 1982, 41 percent of Catholic hospitals (228 of total universe) had ethics committees and 19 percent of the survey respondents listed decision making as a function, and comparable but incomplete figures for 1983 show 50 percent (247) with committees with 11 percent fulfilling a decision making role. This constant growth pattern suggests that Catholic hospitals are leaders in the field and that educational and policy-development activities are still their major orientation.

Nonetheless, the future of ethics committees in Catholic health care cannot be predicted with accuracy. For example, the role of decision making in specific cases of ethical importance may be eliminated in most institutions because it could create liability for committee members and obscure the final responsibility of the physician in charge of patient's care. The advisory and consultative role of committees does not, of course, create these problems.

Notes

1. 366 A, 2d. 641, New Jersey Supreme Court, 1976.

2. Sr. Joan Kalchbrenner, Sr. Margaret John Kelly, Donald G. McCarthy, "Ethics Committees and Ethicists in Catholic Hospitals," *Hospital Progress* (September 1983), pp. 47-51.

3. Kalchbrenner, Kelly, and McCarthy, p. 47.

4. Stuart Youngner, "A National Survey of Hospital Ethics Committees" (Appendix F), in *Deciding to Forego Life-Sustaining Treatment: Ethical, Medical and Legal Issues in Treatment Decisions* (Washington, DC: U.S. Government Printing Office, 1983), pp. 443-457.

5. Youngner, p. 446.

Part Two
Contemporary Context: Issues Facing Ethics Committees

The Church As Teacher

Most Rev. Daniel E. Pilarczyk

Abp. Pilarczyk distinguishes between law and teaching and magisteria and explains the connection between the Ethical and Religious Directives for Catholic Health Facilities and the teaching Church. These Directives are rules for moral conduct derived from the Church's understanding of biblical revelation about human persons and their rights and responsibilities to themselves and one another. Ethics committees in Catholic health facilities respond to the Church's teaching role as they apply the Directives to institutional policy and particular situations.

At some time in his or her life, every Catholic has said, implicitly or explicitly, "I believe all the truths that the Holy Catholic Church believes and teaches." This is, in part at least, an act of faith, a basic commitment to Christ's Church and in virtue of which we call ourselves Catholics. Also, at some time, every person involved with Catholic health care has said or heard said, implicitly or explicitly, "There will be no ghost surgery performed in this facility, because we are a Catholic hospital and such a practice is contrary to the *Ethical and Religious Directives for Catholic Health Facilities.*" My purpose in this chapter is to connect those two statements, to demonstrate the connection between the *Directives* and faith, to view the *Directives* in the context of the Church as teacher.

In pursuit of this purpose observations must be made about *what* the Church teaches, *who* teaches in the name of the Church, and *how* the Church's teachers go about their task. After that I will make several distinctions and then address the genesis and purpose of the *Directives* and the role of the local bishop in their

Abp. Pilarczyk is Archbishop of Cincinnati.

implementation. In anticipation of my concluding remarks, I make the standard disclaimer using Thomas Hardy's words:

Much is there waits you we have missed;
Much lore we leave you worth the knowing;
Much, much has lain outside our ken.

What Does the Church Teach?

Let us turn our ken, then, to *what* the Church teaches. Basically and finally the Church exists to be an extension and continuation of the presence of the God-man in the world, to bring his saving presence into every time and every place. The Church's whole purpose is to bring women and men into contact with the person of the Redeemer. One mode of the Church's mission, one aspect of her work, is to teach; that is, to present in some form that can be learned the truths that lead to acceptance of Christ and to membership and activity in his community of believers that we call the Church. As the extension and continuation of the presence of Christ, the Church is called and sent to teach what Christ taught, to be the teacher in Christ's name, to convey his truth and his doctrine. The Church teaches in the name of Christ. This means that what the Church teaches is what Christ teaches. Now, what Christ teaches is found in Scripture—the recorded words of Christ and his immediate followers—and so the Church teaches the same truths that are found in Scripture. Like every book, however, Scripture requires readers and interpretation. Consequently, the teaching of the Church is the truth of Scripture as read by the community of Christ (the Church) down through the centuries, beginning with the context of Old Testament revelation in which Jesus taught and continuing through the Church's lived experience of Christ and his teachings that we call tradition. But the Church is not content with the mere repetition of the words of Jesus and his first followers. When she teaches Christ she also deals with the presumptions of his teaching, with its implications, and with its consequences. Moreover, the Church does not concern itself just with belief (doctrine), but also with behavior (morals).

If someone wants to know specifically what the Church teaches and about what matters she teaches, that person might turn to the highly technical *Enchiridion Symbolorum,* the standard theological collection of Church definitions and declarations on matters of faith and morals gathered by Henry Denzinger. One might also turn to more accessible works like Richard McBrien's *Catholicism* or John Hardon's *The Catholic Catechism.* In the face of these rather weighty volumes, one might be tempted to ask what has happened to the simple truths that Jesus taught his followers: love God, love yourself, love your neighbor. What has happened is that the Church has been praying and reflecting on these truths for two thousand years and has seen that they have implications and consequences that reach from the dogma of the Holy Trinity to the principle of double effect, from the Council of Nicea defining the divinity of Christ to Pope John Paul II writing about the rights of labor unions. The Church has some teaching about practically everything, because the reality of Christ touches practically everything. Who Teaches in the Name of the Church?

Who, then, teaches in the name of the Church? To whom do we turn to find out what teachings are Christ's teachings, what teachings are in accord with and consequential to what he taught? Jesus gave the responsibility to teach to his apostles ("The Eleven") as he came to the end of his earthly existence (Mt. 28:19; Mk. 16:16; Lk. 24:48). Over and over, St. Paul claims as his teaching authority the fact that he is an apostle (Rm. 1:1; 1 Co. 1:1; 2 Co. 1:1; Ga. 1:1; Ep. 1:1; Col. 1:1). The Second Vatican Council, reflecting Church tradition, sees the succession of the collectivity of the apostles in the college of bishops in union with the pope:

> The order of bishops is the successor to the college of the apostles in teaching authority and pastoral rule; or, rather, in the episcopal order the apostolic body continues without a break. (*Lumen Gentium,* 22)

The Council then goes on to say:

> [Bishops] are authentic teachers, that is, teachers endowed with the authority of Christ, who preach to the people committed to them the faith they must believe and put into practice... Bishops, teaching in communion with the Roman Pontiff, are to be respected by all as witnesses to divine and Catholic truth. In matters of faith and morals, the bishops speak in the name of Christ and the faithful are to accept their teaching and adhere to it with a religious assent of soul. This religious submission of will and of mind must be shown in a special way to the authentic teaching authority of the Roman Pontiff, even when he is not speaking *ex cathedra.* (*Lumen Gentium,* 25)

The apostles, then, were constituted the teachers in the Church, and the bishops in union with the pope today exercise that same apostolic function of teaching.

Obviously, they are not the only teachers. Teaching is also provided in the Church by university professors of theology, by teachers in Catholic schools, by CCD teachers, by priests, and by parents. Such teaching, however, is Catholic only to the extent that it is in accord with the Church's official teaching as witnessed by the pope and the bishops. They, and they alone, are the touchstone of right teaching in the Church. That is why the bishop controls the priests' and deacons' faculty to preach. That is why the certification of catechists takes place through the agency of the bishop's chancery. That is why the new Code of Canon Law calls for a mandate from the local bishop for teachers of Catholic theology in Catholic colleges and universities. Many people teach in the Church, but the basic teachers of all are the pope and the bishops. How do the Church's Teachers Teach?

How do the pope and the bishops teach? I wish to answer this question from three different perspectives.

Specific Means. First, popes and bishops use specific means to teach, e.g., conciliar definitions, *ex cathedra* teachings (the pope), encyclical letters (the pope) or pastoral letters (the bishops), ordinary preaching, and administrative decisions or directives about what must or must not be taught or done under the aegis of the Catholic Church. These are some of the means that the teaching authority of the Church employs to carry out its magisterial responsibility.

Degrees of Authority. Second, what are the degrees of authority that various teachings enjoy? Are all teachings of equal weight? No. Some teachings are presented specifically as infallible, as so important to Christian life that the Church puts the whole weight of her authority from Christ behind them and specifically guarantees that they cannot be wrong. Conciliar definitions would fall under this rubric, as would dogma such as the Immaculate Conception of Mary. There are other matters that the Church has taught—always and everywhere—that are part and parcel of the Christian tradition. These matters may not have been specifically defined, but they are so much a part of Christian life that to reject them would imply a rejection of the whole tradition. Among such matters I would include the Church's teaching about the efficacy of prayer and the immorality of perjury. There is also the ordinary exercise of teaching authority on the part of a pope writing in an encyclical to the universal Church. Even though this last is not formally infallible, it must still be accepted, as Vatican II has said, "with religious submission of will and mind." There are, then, various degrees of solemnity with which the Church teaches. Not everything that the Church teaches is taught with equal weight; not everything is dogmatically infallible. That does not mean that everything not solemnly defined is therefore up for grabs, however. It all calls for respectful hearing because it comes from the Church's official teachers.

Determining Teachings. Third, how do bishops determine what to teach? First, the pope and the bishops are not free to make arbitrary decisions about Church teaching. Vatican II is quite clear about that:

> This teaching office is not above the word of God, but serves it, teaching only what has been handed on, listening to it devoutly, guarding it scrupulously, and explaining it faithfully by divine commission and with the help of the Holy Spirit; it draws from this one deposit of faith everything which it presents for belief as divinely revealed.
> (*Dei Verbum,* 10)

The pope and bishops are subject to and limited by the gospel (Scripture) and by previous Church teaching (tradition), both of which "form one sacred deposit of the word of God." This means that any formal teaching implies a process of discernment on the teacher's part, a process that includes at least some elements such as prayer, study of Scripture, study of doctrinal history, examination of the experience of the faithful, and consultation of theological experts. This kind of discernment, in varying degrees of intensity, takes place every time official Church teaching takes place.

Once this discernment has reached an appropriate conclusion, the teacher offers his teaching. In so doing, the teacher decides something—that is, the teacher *decides* what is to be taught as Church teaching. The pope and bishops, according to circumstances, determine to what the Church will lend her teaching authority; in other words, the pope and the bishops determine what the Church will "certify" as being in accord with Christ's teaching. Sometimes such a decision will deal with that which the faithful must necessarily believe if they wish to remain members of the Church; sometimes such a decision will determine that which the faithful *may* believe or do without fear of contradicting the Gospel. In any case, the process of official Church teaching always seems to include both discernment and decision.

Distinctions in Teaching

Before I proceed to some consideration of the *Ethical and Religious Directives,* I would like to comment on two sets of distinctions. The first distinction is between teaching and law. In its simplest form, law is a prescription for behavior in society. Thus, for example, a person earning a certain salary must pay a certain income tax. In civil society, laws are relatively easy to change; it takes only a majority of legislators to do so. The content of laws is determined by what legislators think is best in the given circumstances, or, more exactly in the existential context, by what the legislators can agree on.

Teaching, on the other hand, is a pronouncement about what the teacher believes to be true. Teaching is determined by what is, or, more exactly, by what the teacher has discerned to be. Ideally, teaching is a true reflection of reality. Teaching can be changed only by persuading the teacher that the teaching is not true or that it is capable of better and more precise formulation.

The Church has both laws and teachings as well as an intermediate area in which the two overlap. For example, Church authority has promulgated a law that says that when someone is appointed bishop of a diocese, he must take possession of his see within two months. The law could say within ten days or within six months, but it says two months. It depends on the legislator's will. On the other hand, the Church teaches that the faculty of speech in human beings has a social dimension and is therefore not under the individual's arbitrary determination. This is a conclusion that the Church has drawn from Christ's teachings. It is not the result of an arbitrary legislative decision. In between these two lies what we call the Church's moral law, which says, for example, do not tell lies. These so-called moral laws are really the pragmatic conclusions of basic Christian teaching and are not laws at all if by law we mean a legislative determination. They are, rather, teachings expressed in the form of precept, or, more exactly, precepts based immediately on Church teaching. The National Conference of Catholic Bishops' *Ethical and Religious Directives* are laws only in this sense; they are rules of moral conduct immediately derived from Christian moral teaching. The *Directives* do not exist because somebody decided that that is the way things should be, but because somebody in teaching authority discerned that such is the implication of Christ's teaching and chose to express that teaching in the form of a rule or precept.

I once heard a lawyer ask what the process would be to change the Church's law on contraception; there was a lengthy discussion. It could have been very brief if someone had only pointed out that the "law" about contraception is much less law than teaching; and that a change involves persuading the teacher that the practical conclusion of *Humanae Vitae* is susceptible of a better formulation or is not in accord with the teaching of Christ, which is exactly what the majority of the commission established by Pope Paul VI was unable to do.

Distinction in Magisteria

The second distinction that I would like to discuss is one that has arisen in the past few years between the magisterium of the bishops and the magisterium of the theologians. I happen to believe that this is not a useful distinction because it seems to imply that there are two teaching authorities in the Church, bishops and theologians, and that people are free to choose which magisterium they will follow. Vatican II and the Church's tradition are clear about who speaks for the Church and about where the Church's teaching authority lies. Nonetheless, the distinction is probably destined to remain with us for a while, and so I think it might be useful to define how I, at least, would describe each.

The *episcopal magisterium,* on the one hand, is the teaching role of the bishops in union with the pope as official spokesmen for the Church. This teaching authority is directed toward all members of the Church and has as its object the acceptance of the proposed teaching in the context of faith. This magisterium depends for its authority on the authority of both Christ and his Church.

The teaching power of theologians, the *theological magisterium,* on the other hand, is primarily concerned with the professional academic activity of theologians. It involves investigation and exploration of the implications of Christ's teaching and is directed primarily toward other theologians for reaction, response, and testing. It is not a pastoral activity but a scientific one and depends for its authority on the validity of the argumentation that is presented.

When people confuse these two, they get themselves into trouble. They tend to condition their assent to what the pope and bishops teach according to the cogency of the argumentation alone, without regard to teaching authority. On the other hand, they tend to judge the value of theologians' teaching on the basis of popular acceptance rather than according to strict academic standards. Thus we hear the response: "No matter how many bishops say it, I must be convinced. If enough theologians say it, it must be true."

This is not to say that the theologians have nothing to contribute to Church teaching. On the contrary, their role is important, indeed essential, in the process of discernment of what is in accord with Christ's teachings. The final responsibility of determining what will be offered as Church teaching, however, remains that of the episcopal magisterium alone, that is, the bishops in union with the pope. Both roles are necessary, but they are different, and the people of God are ill served if the roles are confused.

Ethical Directives

An unofficial code of ethics was proposed by the Catholic Hospital Association (CHA) in 1920 and published in the first issue of Hospital Progress. This code was a reprint of the "Surgical Code for Catholic Hospitals for the Diocese of Detroit," which had been prepared by Fr. M.P. Bourke. Beginning in July 1946, CHA began to press its bishops' representatives for a revised code. This resulted eventually in the appointment by CHA's executive committee of Fr. Gerald Kelly, SJ, to prepare such a code. This code was finished by 1948 and received wide acceptance. In 1954 this code was approved by the bishops of the United States as their official medical code, subject to the approval of the local ordinaries for use in their dioceses.

By 1967, the medical as well as the ecclesial situation had undergone considerable evolution, and in November 1967 the

Commission on Church Health Services was established by the United States Catholic Conference (USCC) to study problems arising from the medical-moral code. This commission received recommendations from the Catholic Theological Society of America and in 1969 submitted a request to the USCC's administrative committee that the code then in force be revised by an appropriate agency of the bishops' conference. Eventually this task was assigned to the conference's Department of Health Affairs in conjunction with the Committee on Doctrine. CHA kept urging the bishops' conference to complete its work; the code was approved at the bishops' meeting in November 1971 as a national code, although it remained up to each bishop to apply it in his own diocese. Some theologians reacted to certain parts of the code; some physicians counterreacted. Eventually several questions arising from the code on tubal ligation and material cooperation were presented to the Holy See, and the Roman response together with a commentary was published in 1977. Although some of the code was revised in 1975, the code today is basically the code that was approved by the bishops in 1971.

What is it, then, that exists in the present *Ethical and Religious Directives?* It is a compilation of Church teachings on certain specific moral questions arising from a request for direction from the health care community and arrived at by the bishops through a discernment process that included suggestions and reactions from the theological and medical communities. The *Directives* are in the form of rules or regulations, but they are basically proximate reflections of teachings that are proposed with the authority of the Church's teachers and ultimately rooted in the Gospel. It is true that the application of the *Directives* at the local level depends on the diocesan bishop. This is due, I believe, to a technicality, namely, that the bishops' conference does not have the authority to teach officially. This is the responsibility of each individual bishop. This is not to say, however, that the local bishop is free to pick and choose among the directives or is free to reject them totally. The *Directives* reflect the ordinary teachings of the Church that Church members are obliged to accept and that local bishops are responsible for upholding and fostering. The local bishop is also charged with interpreting the code and directing its application in specific situations that arise in his diocese. Here again, the bishop is not free to accept or reject the basic teaching, since the teaching reflects the teaching of the Church universal. His task as interpreter is to make a prudent judgment on how the *Directives* fit into the complexities of individual situations that arise in Catholic health care facilities in his jurisdiction. He exercises this responsibility not as hospital administrator or as rulemaker, but as spokesman for the Church's teachings.

In this context I must say something about what is called "geographic morality," the situation in which a bishop of one diocese permits or tolerates medical procedures that a neighboring bishop does not. It is essential to note that what is at issue here is not necessarily a doctrinal rejection of one or more of the *Directives.* The *Directives* reflect standard Catholic teaching, which bishops are pledged to support and promulgate. What is at issue is the application of moral principles to the complexities of a local situation. This is what is called a prudential judgment. One weighs the principles against the situation and makes the best decision possible while respecting the demands of both. This is not always easy. Two prudent persons can conceivably come up with different responses to the same set of problems if the problems are sufficiently complex. Likewise, situations that appear similar may actually differ from one place to another and the same prudent man might come up with different responses to each. What we must remember is that we are dealing with highly specific situations that affect a small number of persons under Catholic health care. Quite frankly, I would like to see more uniformity in some of the judgments that are allegedly made, but at the same time I am not in a position to say that every decision that differs from what I would have decided is wrong.

Conclusion

Let us now conclude by going back to the point at which we began. When health care personnel hear someone say, "There will be no ghost surgery performed in this facility because we are a Catholic hospital, and such a practice is contrary to the *Ethical and Religious Directives for Catholic Health Facilities,*" they are hearing a statement about a Christian view of human personhood. They are hearing a statement about the Church's teaching authority. They are hearing a statement about what the Holy Catholic Church believes and teaches. They are hearing a statement about Christ and about faith.

Discussion After Archbishop Pilarczyk's Lecture

Question: What should be the Church's attitude today toward contemporary ethicists outside the Judeo-Christian tradition? How do we avoid a ghetto mentality?

Abp. Pilarczyk: What you are asking is basically the question of the relationship between philosophy and revelation. As we all know, there is no one simple answer to that. Obviously, human insights are useful in enriching and elaborating on some of the implications of the Gospel. The fact remains, however, that the Gospel stands in judgment on human philosophy and that we cannot allow ourselves to say that if there is enough pressure from human philosophy we must give way. Our faith teaches us that, no matter how much pressure there is from human philosophy, there are certain points on which we must not give way. The danger of the ghetto mentality arises when we do not even want to hear what human philosophy has to say. I view that as a highly defensive posture, one of enclosure. The Gospel has nothing to fear from human philosophy. The Gospel stands in judgment on it even though it can also be enriched by it.

Question: Archbishop, what do you say about a statement such as the following that might be applied to not only an individual, but also to a Catholic hospital that, in general, at least, has accepted the *Ethical and Religious Directives:* "There is a Christian right to dissent conscientiously in practice from reformable Church teaching and pastoral directives."

Abp. Pilarczyk: The question that is inherent in the difficulty that you raise is, "Who speaks for the Church?" I think that the ecclesiology of Vatican II is quite clear about who can commit the Church's authority to a given teaching: it is the bishops in union with the pope. I think that dissent stands in the category of the discernment process. It is not inappropriate for theologians and other qualified persons to take issue with a teaching in the hope of making it more perfect, in the hope of making it more clear, in the hope of teasing out its implications a little more extensively. But it seems to me that that is all in the discernment process.

The decision-making process about what the Church teaches and about what the Church asks in the context of behavior from its members is the bishops' province and responsibility. Consequently,

I think that those who believe they have a *right* to dissent in practice from the Church's teachings are saying that it is up to them to decide which teachings they will choose to carry out in practice. To say that anyone in the Church has a right to dissent in practice from what the Church teaches is simply to say that everybody has a right to disobey what the Church teaches. If that is the case, the Church's teaching authority becomes virtually nonexistent.

Question: I do not understand the difference between prudential judgment and situation ethics.

Abp. Pilarczyk: According to traditional Catholic moral teaching, in any moral decision that we make, we are trying to apply a principle to a concrete situation. For example, we are supposed to pay our debts. But, if I receive a credit card bill that includes an interest charge that I have not incurred, must I pay that interest? The principle is that you must pay your *just* debts. The situation here is that I have a bill that is not just or that I perceive to be unjust, and therefore I make out a check for an amount less that undue interest. Traditional Catholic moral teaching is always about that tension between principle and circumstances. You cannot have a moral judgment that does not include circumstances.

The difference between what I have just described and situation ethics, is that situation ethics tends to say that there never is a situation in which a principle must necessarily be applied, or, more exactly, that no principles are unchangeable in every situation. The difference, basically, is that with a prudential judgment you are trying to unite two things, principle and situation, and keep them both—to respond to the needs of the situation and to maintain the principle. Situation ethics tends to put the emphasis on the context and say that the needs of the context or the situation are the primary determining factors. Those who follow Catholic moral teaching also maintain the principle.

Question: One of the questions that comes to us frequently is the fact that, as a Catholic hospital—and the only hospital in the area —we are said to be imposing our morality on others. Could you comment on this, please?

Abp. Pilarczyk: Catholic health care does not exist primarily to provide every kind of health care to every person. Catholic health care exists primarily as a witness to the Church's reality, as a witness to Church teaching, as a witness to the love of Christ for his people in the context of sickness and wellness. If we believe that certain procedures or practices are in disaccord with the law of the Gospel and with the law of the love of Christ for his people, to cooperate in such procedures or practices is to give counterwitness to the love of Christ. In doing what is wrong we harm ourselves and the people whom we wrong. Therefore, it is quite consistent and quite moral and quite responsible for a Catholic hospital to say that it exists for certain purposes, among which is health care, but also among which is witness to the Gospel of Christ as we believe it. If others come to us and want us to do things that we believe are contrary to the Gospel law of Christ, they ask us to be false to our reason for being. To say that a Catholic hospital has a conscience of its own is simply to say that a Catholic hospital is not the same as other hospitals. Therefore, it is not inappropriate for a Catholic hospital to be true to its conscience. It is not imposing anything on anybody. If a local civic community thinks it wants more and different procedures than the Catholic hospital can provide, it has the right to say to the Catholic hospital, "Either you must leave or you must stop being Catholic." And the Catholic hospital has the right to say, "We will not stop being Catholic; if the only other option is to leave, we will leave." We must be careful about other people's consciences, but we must be careful about our own, too.

Question: Very complex things are happening in health care today, and the direct care providers, such as the pediatricians and the nurses, who are really caught in the hard vise of these decisions, desperately need the best assistance for discernment that can be provided. But there are not enough theologians or philosophers available to us out there in the vineyard to do the kinds of things that you are talking about today.

Abp. Pilarczyk: You make an excellent and important point, but I would like to point out that, superficial as this sounds, expert authority and guidance for a specific situation is only as far away as the telephone. This is where groups like CHA and the Pope John XXIII Medical-Moral Research and Education Center provide a valuable service to the Church.

Ethical Methodologies:
A Current Controversy

Benedict Ashley, OP

Fr. Ashley analyzes the current controversy over exceptionless moral norms within Catholic moral theology because members of ethics committees need to deal with such norms. While recognizing the weakness of a legalistic approach to the moral law, Fr. Ashley also offers serious objections to the new approach of some Catholic ethicists called proportionalism. He points out that ethics committees in Catholic facilities are expected to uphold the Church's exceptionless opposition to such practices as abortion, euthanasia, and contraceptive sterilization.

Rather than deal with the range of current ethical methodologies extending from situationism to legalism, it may be more profitable to concentrate on the principal point of controversy that at present divides Catholic moral theologians, namely, the validity of what is generally called "proportionalism" as a method of making moral decisions. My aim is to present both sides of this controversy, but I will not conceal my own opposition to proportionalism. It is a controversy that I hope can be resolved through fair and frank theological discussion without the intervention of the magisterium.

Even before Vatican II, most Catholic theologians were convinced that the type of moral theology formerly taught in Catholic schools and seminaries according to the approach developed after the Council of Trent was seriously inadequate; it did not lack merit, but it failed to root Christian morality in fundamental Christian doctrine. Instead, this so-called manual moral theology presented Christian life simply as obedience to the law, rather than as transformation by the Gospel. To accuse this type of moral

Fr. Ashley, OP, is professor of Moral Theology, Aquinas Institute, St. Louis, MO.

theology of legalism is not to deny the necessary role of law—natural, positive, ecclesiastical, and divine—in the moral life but to insist that law is only an instrument of and not the source of Christian morality. Yet manual moral theology tended to stay at the superficial level of legality and to reduce morality to obedience to the laws of God, Church, and state in view of rewards and punishments.

Such a morality by the manual runs the danger of minimalism: How far can I go without breaking the law? That attitude is still operative frequently in Catholic medical-ethical decisions. Hospitals and physicians want to know: How far can we go without violating the *Ethical and Religious Directives for Catholic Health Facilities?* To think in this way is to see law as an obstacle to action rather than as a means to more effective action. Hence we might find a hospital trying to solve its ethical dilemmas by wheeling the patient to a nearby non-Catholic hospital for procedures forbidden to Catholic hospitals by the *Directives.* The traditional moral theology unintentionally fostered this kind of hypocrisy by its mechanical rigidity. Laws necessarily resist modification and thus soon appear obsolete in the face of new problems. This gap between law and reality soon breeds contempt for the law. Because everyone naturally resents arbitrary restrictions on legitimate freedom, we all rebel against and attempt to void regulations that appear unreasonable. This resentment against the Church's magisterial teaching from health care professionals appears in their question: Why does the Church impose these limitations on our expert efforts to bring the best kind of medical care to our patients?

Magisterial Teaching/Public Opinion Gap

Most moral theologians today are keenly aware of this gap between magisterial teaching and public and professional opinion. Thus it is generally agreed that this gap cannot be closed without a profound revision of ethical methodology. The disagreement is not over that necessity but over what direction this revision should take. One proposal seems to dominate most publications in this field and is widely influential in schools of theology, seminaries, and even in catechetical instruction. Unquestionably it effected a great change in the practice of pastoral counseling. It seems to appeal especially to the pragmatic, psychologizing turn of American culture and is thus plausible and attractive to many. Although it originated with distinguished European moralists such as Joseph Fuchs, Peter Knauer, and Bruno Schüler, it has able proponents in Richard McCormick and Charles Curran (although Curran has formulated it differently as a "theology of compromise), undoubtedly the two best known and widely respected Catholic moral theologians in the United States. One of the chief reasons for its success is that many suppose that the only alternative is a return to the sterile legalism that I have described, and it is in terms of this harsh dichotomy between the old and the new, the traditional and the progressive, the "classic but static" and the "historical and dynamic," that is the legalistic and the personalistic, that the controversy too often is framed.

Nature of Proportionalism

In a brief summary it is not possible to do full justice to the proportionalists' case, which in the course of the controversy has become very nuanced, but the essence of the method can be made clear. First, proportionalism is *not* "situationism." Situation ethics as developed by Joseph Fletcher reduced all moral norms to a single principle—"do what is most loving." Proportionalism, on the contrary, accepts the validity of moral norms as *prima facie* guides to moral decision making. The moral norms traditional to Catholicism and characteristic of the better elements of U.S. culture are assumed as the point of departure for ethical reflection. Thus, I know of no proportionalist writer who denies that the Ten Commandments or the Sermon on the Mount contain the fundamental norms of Christian morality. Nor is proportionalism a "subjectivist" morality, because it insists that moral reflection must consider not only the affective attitudes of the subjects but all ascertainable objective aspects, notably the practical consequences of acts and their effects on both persons and the environment.

What characterizes proportionalism is the method it employs in applying moral norms to concrete decisions, especially when these decisions involve a conflict of norms. In such cases, the question arises whether authentic morality permits, or even demands, that an exception to concrete moral norms be made in order not to sacrifice the good of human persons to a merely mechanical application of the law (legalism). Was it not precisely against such legalism on the part of the scribes and Pharisees that Jesus indignantly said, "The Sabbath was made for man, and not man for the Sabbath" (Mk. 2:27)?

Traditional moral theology admitted that in conflict situations exceptions sometimes must be made in order to obey a *higher* moral norm (e.g., the norm "Thou shalt not kill" does not apply when it conflicts with the higher norm of self-defense or the preservation of justice for society). In such cases the criteria of "proportion" between an act's good and bad consequences was an important consideration. Clearly, to justify an exception to a *prima facie* valid norm, it is necessary to show that this exception will result in a greater good or will avoid a greater evil. Catholic moral theology, however (and this is the crucial point), has traditionally always maintained that some (even if very few) concrete moral norms are so fundamental that they never can permit exception, there are, in other words, no higher moral norms to which appeal can be made to justify these exceptions. One of these is "Thou shalt not kill the innocent (e.g., a nonaggressor)." Reference has commonly been made to the heinous immorality of Caiphas' argument for the death of Jesus even if he be innocent, "Can you not see that it is better for you to have one man die than to have the whole nation destroyed?" (Jn. 11:50) Such negative and exceptionless norms are said to be against actions that are *per se malum* (intrinsically evil).

Proportionalists have often stated their case by saying that no one has ever satisfactorily shown why or how it is possible to classify some *kinds* of acts (i.e., a type of act defined in the abstract) as intrinsically evil. Hence, they have said, it is necessary to find some more secure method of moral decision than to fall back on such an undemonstrated foundation. It would seem, they suggest, that moralists have been so confident of declaring that certain kinds of acts are intrinsically immoral because they were relying on the essentially platonic notion that we can deduce an act's morality or immorality from its conformity or nonconformity with an abstract idea or definition of "human nature." Modern philosophy, science, and biblical exegesis do not support this misplaced confidence, since all these disciplines have made us aware of the essential historicity of human nature, which must forever remain a mystery that gradually reveals itself in our historical experiences rather than a static essence totally transparent to our inspection. More recently, however, proportionalists have clarified their position by admitting that they too concede the existence of some moral norms that are exceptionless when stated in a sufficiently abstract manner. It is always immoral to hate God or neighbor, for example, because such a norm is so abstract that it does not define what precisely is meant by "hate." Moreover, they point out that it may be possible to state an exceptionless moral norm if we do so in an extremely concrete and particularized formula that includes "value terms." It is always wrong to commit adultery, for example, if by "adultery" is meant an act that does an *injustice* to the other party, because "injustice" is a value term that qualifies the statement enough to render it concrete, rather than abstract, and thus begs the question of moral decision. Evidently, therefore, the essence of proportionalism is not a denial of exceptionless norms as such, although, as I will show, an important consequence of this position is the possibility of affirming exceptions to many of the traditional norms.

Proportionalist Position

The essence of the proportionalists' position is the claim that the ultimate criterion for all moral decisions is the proportion of premoral value and disvalue that the act will evoke. Is not this principle self-evident, since it would seem that to deny it is to affirm that an act can be moral even if it will probably do more harm than good? What might seem obscure in this principle is the term "premoral value and disvalue." Why not just say "the proportion of good and evil"? The answer, of course, is that if we were to say that it is permissible to perform an act that was more good than evil, it still would be evil according to the ancient maxim that "an act, to be morally good, must be good in all respects," This maxim rests on the fact that morality ultimately resides in the righteous will of the agent, who cannot intend both good and evil simultaneously. Jesus taught this when he said, "What emerges from within a man, that and nothing else is what makes him impure (Mk. 7:20). Nor do proportionalists wish to fall under the condemnation of St. Paul, who rejected the notion that "we may do evil that good may come of it" (Rm. 3.8) or the old canard of advocating that "the end justifies the means." Consequently, proportionalists maintain that in moral decisions the proportion to be ascertained is not between *moral* evil and *moral* good but between *premoral* values, positive and negative. Only after this proportion has been determined can the act be judged morally good (if the values outweigh the disvalues) or morally evil (if the disvalues outweigh the values). Thus, proportionalists will never do what is morally evil in order to achieve a greater good; they will only do an act that, though it involves some harm, accomplishes a greater benefit.

In assaying this proportion of values and disvalues foreseen as the effects of a given act, proportionalists claim that they take into account, just as did traditional moralists, not only the agent's intention and the act's circumstances (as would a situationist), but also the act's intrinsic nature (the "moral object," in traditional terminology) in its relation to the person and the person's transcendent destiny. Nevertheless, in considering all three of these criteria, the proportionalists deny that the nature of the act (on which *prima facie* norms are based) absolutely determines the act's morality or immorality, since this depends on the proportion of *all* the values and disvalues involved, some of which arise from intention or circumstances and may thus outweigh the act's *prima facie* immorality. Thus, proportionalists are ready to admit exceptions to abstract moral norms in many instances where traditional moralists have excluded them because the act, by its very nature, apart from intention and circumstances, is intrinsically evil.

The seeming practical advantages of the proportionalist method as a way to solve conflict situations should now be clear. Whereas legalism had made it appear that Catholic morality insists on a rigid, inhuman, heartless, and pharasaic application of moral norms, proportionalism shows how to apply these same *prima facie* valid norms in such a way that even in difficult conflicts care is always taken to maximize the benefit to persons and minimize the unavoidable harm.

Inadequacy of Proportionalism

The supposed merit of proportionalism is that it enables us to solve difficult conflicts without lapsing into mere situationism, while, at the same time, maintaining the general validity of Christian moral norms and thus avoiding cultural relativism. The objections that have now been raised by a considerable number of philosophers (Elizabeth Anscombe and Germain Grisez) and moralists (Frederick Carney and Paul Ramsey among Protestant ethicists and William May and Servais Pinckaers among Catholic moralists) are of several sorts, but all center on the contention that proportionalism as a practical system of moral decision making is impractical because it inevitably leads to arbitrary judgments that ultimately depend on the prejudices or cultural conditioning of the persons making such decisions.

One way of raising this objection is to point out that it is difficult to distinguish this supposedly new methodology from the familiar theories of consequentialism and utilitarianism. Consequentialism holds that the criterion of an act's morality is the balance of good consequences over evil consequences foreseen as the act's probable results. Utilitarianism agrees with this criterion but also proposes to calculate this proportion by a kind of quantitative estimation of the relative goodness and evil of the consequences. Since philosophers have pretty well exposed these system's weaknesses, proportionalists are quick to distinguish their system from consequentialism—on the grounds that they take into account not only an act's consequences, but its intrinsic values— and from utilitarianism—on the grounds that they weigh values qualitatively as well as quantitatively. Whether these distinctions are more than verbal is not clear because no proportionalist whom I have read ever explains just how this weighing is made, except by referring vaguely to a "hierarchy of values," to "common estimation," or to intuitive "gut feelings." If proportionalism is to be accepted as a valid new method, it must explain more precisely how to proportion values and disvalues.

The answer usually given to this demand is that the traditional methodology often spoke of "proportion" and never explained very clearly how it was to be ascertained. Weaknesses in the traditional methodology, however, are hardly strengths in the new one. In any case, John Connery has well answered this excuse by showing that the conception of "proportion did not play an essential role in the traditional methodology, since it was merely used as a sign that something might be wrong with a moral decision that seemed to result in more harm than good, rather than as the essential determinant of morality or immorality. It is indeed self-evident that it cannot be moral to act in a way that intentionally produces more harm than good. Since, however, what is "good" for persons includes what is "morally good" for them, it begs the question to try to determine what is most beneficial for them on the basis of premoral values and disvalues.

This brings me to what I believe is the fundamental argument against proportionalism and to what reveals its essentially arbitrary character. I maintain that *proportionalism is self-contradictory* and can be used to justify or condemn any act whatsoever. Proportionalists admit that if the proportion in question was a weighing of the moral goods against the moral evils involved in an act, the method would justify doing evil so that good might come from it, namely, "justifying the means by the end." Thus, they would have to admit that it is permissible to kill 1 million innocent persons if by doing so one could save the lives of 1 million and one innocent persons, or it would be permissible for a soldier ordered to rape a woman to do so to save his own life (because rape is a lesser moral evil than murder). Consequently, they reject any such calculus of moral goods and evils and determine the proportion only by a calculus of *premoral* values and disvalues. This reasoning, however, results in a self-contradiction; it implies that these values are at the same time premoral and moral. That these values be premoral is required lest proportionalism justify doing evil that good may come from it, but they must simultaneously be moral or they cannot be weighed to determine their proportion.

This latter half of the contradiction becomes evident if we actually attempt to carry out the weighing process. In order to determine that one premoral value is less, equal to, or greater than another, it must, as the proportionalists themselves admit, be ranked in a "hierarchy of values." But what determines this ranking? The term *value* necessarily implies a relation to an end or the end itself; it is valuable *for* something or *in itself.* But if we are speaking of *human* values (and any other kind of values are irrelevant to our problem), this relation is to the supreme value of human life—to the end of human life. Yet an act considered as the goal of human life or as a means relative to that goal is precisely what we mean by a *moral* value. Thus, premoral values can be measured to determine their proportion only if they are moral values—obviously a contradiction.

Why have the proportionalists not recognized this self-contradiction in their own position? I believe the answer can be found in the fact that there is an historical link between proportionalism and the ethical system of the phenomenological philosopher Max Scheler, who taught that values are phenomenological essences of a special kind that in the abstract are known *intuitively* in an absolute mode and that can be realized concretely in human life only imperfectly. It is questionable whether this intuitionist and ultimately idealistic philosophy of ethics is compatible with Christian realism. What is certain is that, as embodied in the current proportionalism, it leads to a contradiction. The result is that when we look at the actual ethical positions proportionalists take in the current literature, especially the medical-ethical literature, we find that they come to a variety of conclusions about whether and when abortion, sterilization, contraception, euthanasia, and various kinds of extramarital sex are permissible exceptions to *prima facie* moral norms. These various estimates of the values and disvalues of particular acts seem largely to be the result of the ethicist's ingenuity and imagination in discovering a longer list of values than of disvalues for acts approved by our secular culture and, conversely, for those popularly disapproved. Thus the role of Christian ethics as a witness to the Kingdom of God standing in prophetic judgment on "the ways of the world" collapses.

It is no wonder that proportionalism has been advocated chiefly by writers who have adopted a position of "dissent" with respect to certain of the moral teachings of the magisterium, particularly those of *Humanae Vitae.* The magisterium seems stubbornly committed to the view that there are absolute, exceptional, and *concrete* moral norms, such as that abortion and contraceptive sterilization are always wrong. Proportionalists are also faced with the apparent inconsistency of some of their conclusions with the absoluteness of biblical moral norms, and they attempt to solve this difficulty by the rather desperate argument that the biblical teachings should be understood not as normative, but merely as *paranetic,* that is, exhortations to do good but empty of any permanently valid instruction on what is good or bad. Thus, "Thou shall not commit adultery" would mean for us today, "Do not commit a sexual sin," meaning by "sexual sin" whatever in today's culture is regarded as a "sexual sin."

An Alternative to Proportionalism

Proportionalism seems to have gained wide support chiefly because the only alternative known to many is the legalism of the manuals. It is notable that proportionalism, in its opposition to legalism, does not make a radical break with the preoccupation of the post-Tridentine moral theology with the solution of conflicts. Historians of moral theology have shown that in the late Middle Ages Christian ethics shifted from a sapiential approach to morality in terms of the formation of Christian character by the infused and acquired virtues and the restoration of the image of God in the human person in the likeness of Jesus Christ to a voluntaristic and therefore legalistic ethics centered on cases of conscience. Proportionalist ethical theory remains within that voluntaristic tradition, since the kind of questions it raises are largely confined to solving conflicts between moral rules.

The alternative to proportionalism, therefore, is not legalism, but a radical break with legalism and a return to a way of viewing moral questions more in line with an older and more continuous tradition of Christian moral thinking, one more securely rooted in Christian anthropology. The starting point for such a moral theory is not philosophical but theological and consists in the interrelation between four biblical themes: (1) the human person is created in God's image; (2) this image is restored through God's offering himself to us in the Old and New Covenant; (3) the New Covenant, through which God's image is perfectly restored, is found in Jesus Christ, the Incarnate Word, and (4) this restoration is effected by the power of Christ's Holy Spirit. *Thus, the supreme moral norm becomes conformity to Christ.* Since in Christ the human and the divine are perfectly united without distortion, this conformity to Christ is at once the perfect fulfillment of our native humanity and the transformation of that humanity by participation in the life of the Trinity.

In this perspective, Christian morality is the fulfillment of God's law, but since that law is the divine wisdom leading us to human restoration and deification in Christ, this morality is not merely conformity to law, but, much more profoundly, it is conformity to Christ. Such conformity does not mean, of course, that our lives become carbon copies of the life of Christ. Each of us was created unique by God and must live out our witness to Christ in his or her own special time and place in history. We imitate Jesus by recovering our true selves as God created us to be, brothers and sisters of Christ, adopted into his company. This conformity means that we share the same common nature, human yet elevated by grace, as that of Jesus Christ. Without that community in being we cannot be members of his companionship, of his kingdom. This common nature would not be common unless it were constituted by certain fundamental needs and capacities, such as the need for bodily health, family life, human society, and knowledge of the world, oneself and other persons, and, above all, of the three divine persons. These basic human needs that unite us to Christ and to the whole human community throughout space and time are the foundation of our relations with one another and of our inalienable human rights. From these rights and the moral obligations to respect these rights arise certain exceptionless moral norms.

Why are these basic moral norms that protect basic human needs and rights exceptionless? Why can violation of these norms and these needs and rights never be morally justified no matter how special the circumstances and no matter what good consequences are anticipated from such a violation? The theological answer is that every human being created in God's image and redeemed by Christ is of unique value and therefore cannot be treated as a mere means to the good of others, even of countless others. We cannot sacrifice the life of the unborn child to enhance the life of its mother, because both are human beings. We cannot destroy the life of one noncombatant in war to save the lives of millions.

Moreover, the human agent in every decision must first of all consider whether he or she is violating his or her own basic need for moral integrity in this act. We cannot lie, even if the lie does no one else harm, or even seems to do them a great deal of good, because it violates our own need to be truthful. We cannot commit an act of sexual impurity, even one of self-abuse or one with another consenting adult to whom we are not committed in marriage, because such acts violate our own sexual integrity. It is the sacredness of the human person in his or her essential constitution as an image of God in Christ that gives an absolute, exceptionless character to basic moral norms. As St. Paul said so graphically, "Do you not see that your bodies are members of Christ? Would you have me take Christ's members and make them the members of a prostitute?" (1 Co. 6:15). What St. Paul says of sexual acts also applies to all Christian acts. They either make us members of Christ and our actions his actions, or they separate us from him. We become what we do.

Does this mean that the Gospel demands a deontological ethics, that is, one based on doing the duties prescribed by law without regard to the consequences, without considering how these acts harm or benefit human beings? By no means. Christian tradition before the late medieval and post-Tridentine turn to voluntarism was always teleological, since it measured the morality of acts by their relation to the goal (*telos*) of union with Christ, and this union with Christ requires us always to love our neighbors, seek their good, and never do them harm. But we can never do good to our neighbor unless we first respect our neighbor's rights, nor can we love others unless we first love ourselves and therefore respect our own moral integrity. The fatal weakness of proportionalism is that it opens the way to the illusion that it is compassionate and realistic to attempt to achieve the human good by violating the basic human rights and obligations when it appears that under certain circumstances this will lead to more good than harm. When a basic human need and right is in question, its violation is always disproportionately harmful, and its protection always outweighs the possible good consequences.

Post-Tridentine moral theology, for all its defects, at least protected this fundamental element of Christian tradition by insisting that some moral laws are absolute. It was better protected by the patristic and scholastic theories of ethics. However, as we revise moral theology today to take better account of modern developments in the understanding of human historicity, depth psychology, sociology, and medical technology, we must include a defense of basic human rights and the exceptionless moral norms that protect them.

Application to Medical Ethics

The proportionalist controversy has arisen mainly in the context of questions in medical ethics regarding contraception and sterilization, abortion, euthanasia, and, recently, artificial reproduction and genetic engineering. Catholic health care facilities are hard pressed by social pressures to permit procedures, at least in hardship cases, that traditionally have been regarded as forbidden by exceptionless moral norms embodied in magisterial documents and in the *Ethical and Religious Directives.* No doubt these norms must be applied with prudence to concrete situations that are sometimes complex and in which the facts of the case are not always easy to ascertain. Moreover, problems of cooperation and of respect for the consciences of others arise. The existence of absolute norms does not imply that our answers to such cases are a cut and dried, mechanical, bureaucratic, and heartless imposition of iron-clad rules. The application, to be prudent, must always be with the honest and careful purpose of fostering the good of all persons involved. The good of human persons is first of all a *moral* good, and we are most compassionate when we make it easier for persons to decide to do what is subjectively and also objectively right, not when we make it easier for them to do what is objectively and perhaps also subjectively wrong.

Conclusion

Thus, in my opinion, for Catholic health care professionals or Catholic health care facilities to adopt the attractive but poorly grounded theory of proportionalism as a method of making medical-moral decisions is shortsighted. They will find that following such a method may at first seem to solve some difficult moral dilemmas. It will permit them to advise contraception and contraceptive sterilization to some women who need to avoid pregnancy, instead of teaching them to use natural family planning effectively. It will permit them to advise abortion in some cases where there "seems no other way out." It may permit them to condone euthanasia in some cases, especially of the defective, the senile, or the comatose to escape heavy burdens of care. It may make them supportive of sex outside marriage for whatever reason. It may even excuse cooperation with some of these once forbidden procedures for the economic good of their family or their institution. But the result will be the gradual, almost hidden erosion of basic human rights and the Christian view of the uniqueness of the person. The change in medical attitudes toward abortion in our lifetime, a change that has for the most part been vigorously opposed by Catholics outside the medical profession rather than by Catholic medical professionals, shows how easily this can happen. Some Catholic theologians, in their reaction to the legalism in which they were educated, have, by their unwise and all too uncritical acceptance of proportionalism, become parties to this tragic conformity to the moral standards of a secular society that talks a great deal about human rights but recognizes no foundation for them other than shifting public opinion.

On the other hand, the way lies open to Catholic health care professionals and Catholic health care facilities, under the guidance of the Holy Spirit and our spiritual shepherds, to be a witness to our sick society of the inviolability of the human person. Moreover, they are called to engage creatively in finding solutions to problems of health care that instead of violating human rights in the name of pragmatic solutions, will promote the full development of human persons in the likeness of Christ.

Discussion After Father Ashley's Lecture

Question: First, I would like a definition from both the proportionalists and their opponents of the nature of a moral act. How does one define a moral act? Then I would like you to illustrate how you define, for instance, a moral act for a group of religious sisters protecting Jewish children from a Gestapo officer who comes and says, "Sister, are the children here?" If she answers, "Yes, the children are here," perhaps 30 children will die. If she answers no, on objective moral terms she's lying.

Fr. Ashley: I do not think that there is any fundamental difference between proportionalists and the people who are criticizing them about the definition of a "moral act." Both agree that a moral act is not merely the physical act of what you do. It is not just killing. For example, if you said, this is an act of killing, that does not make clear whether it is a good or bad moral act. What must also be known is what is *intended* in performing this physical action. The term *intended,* however, means something different to the two groups. When proportionalists talk about the moral object or the nature of the act and the intention and the circumstances, they talk as if there is no intention in the moral act itself. The traditional view of the moral act always implied that there is such an intention; that is what makes it moral. If I intend to perform this act of killing, am I killing an innocent person, killing a criminal, or killing in defense? There is an intention included in the moral act. When you talk traditionally about circumstances and intention as being other factors, this intention in question is some other additional intention. The example ordinarily given is that if I killed an innocent child in order to make money, making the money would be an added intention than the intention of killing the innocent child. The two approaches differ in that aspect.

The example you gave, which is a common one about lying, can be handled in different ways. I think the right way to handle it is by understanding that when we speak in human language it is always in a context. You cannot say what a particular statement means except in context. In this example, the context is obviously one of coercion. Therefore, no matter what was said to the Gestapo officer, it would not be a lie, because any sensible person knows that an answer given under unjust coercion is without meaning, and a statement that is without meaning cannot be a lie. There is no lie in your example.

Question: You talked about cultural relativism, that there is the danger of taking on the norms of a society. I think that in all fairness the proportionalists are saying that our critique of society is the Gospel, our critique comes from the Scriptural values that we find, not leaving aside the basic values that we also find in creation and in the very structure of human life. I think they are saying that each age of the Church must struggle with how to live out these values. Each age is in continuity with the past, but each age also has its own specificity. I do not think the proportionalists are saying they are making these judgments by themselves; it is in the context of the whole faith community that they are making these judgments. As they do that, however, they must embody the Gospel in today's age, so there is a certain factor of culture and history, but it is in continuity with the Church of every age struggling to do that very thing. Finally, you spent most of your time describing what you did not like about the proportionalist school. Could you talk a little bit about what you see as the alternative?

Fr. Ashley: I agree entirely with most of what you said. That is not the point of the controversy. We are all agreed on those things. The question is whether proportionalism really provides a method that can maintain the basic New Testament values. My argument was that because proportionalism is self-contradictory and illogical, it will lead to an erosion of these values. If it is true that proportionalism has this contradictory and arbitrary character, it will not help maintain Christian values.

On the positive side, I certainly would like to enlarge more on what I see as a better moral theology. I think it is sufficient here to say that such a theology must defend our basic human needs and human rights. I do not see how proportionalism can do that because of its abandonment of absolute norms. I think the giveaway is indicated when straight statements in the New Testament that provide for particular norms are brought forward, and proportionalists argue that those norms do not bind us now because they are merely paranetic. If you think of the area of sexual morality, St. Paul is very plain that the only legitimate use of sex is in the context of committed, permanent marriage. Now, is that a matter of God's giving us a specific norm about sexual life, or is that something that is a time-conditioned thing of St. Paul's culture? Is that the way people thought about sex then, but our culture realizes that divorce and homosexuality are permissible? In fact, that is the way the argument develops. The book on human sexuality by the committee of the Catholic Theological Society of America, by explicitly applying the proportionalist method in great detail, ended up advocating a kind of sexual morality that is very close to the current secular view.

Question: I think it is obvious that certain things are culturally conditioned. The Bible says, "Slaves be subject to your masters," and for 1900 years this text was used by many to justify slavery as being based on the Bible. The question is, by what principles in your system would you distinguish those things that are culturally determined and those things that are absolute norms? Is there any basis other than the way we have always done it?

Fr. Ashley: Well, the way we have always done it is not so bad. The view of basic human rights that has generally been held is still very valid. The United Nations produced a document on basic human rights. The Holy See played a big role in developing that document. It has been at least nominally accepted by most of the nations of the world and is a very good statement of what these basic human rights are.

But there is a very real problem. I think it is unfortunate that you can read the whole current literature of moral theology and very little of it has to do with the Scriptures. That was true of the old manual moral theology, too. But I do not really see that proportionalism has contributed to solving that problem. The very crucial example about slavery is a good case in point. If we trace the history of how the Church came to the conviction that there is an absolute prohibition against slavery that St. Paul apparently did not see, that is a very interesting story. Notice, though, that there we are talking about something negative in the New Testament, a lack in the New Testament of seeing all the implications of the principles. That is different from those norms in which the New Testament tells us positively what is right and wrong. And, of course, the interpretation of Scripture as something that has a binding character for Catholics is the work of the magisterium, not of the biblical scholar. The biblical scholars can contribute to it, but they cannot come to the final decision about what the Scriptures mean for our faith and action.

Question: The only way I have been able to deal with seemingly insoluble situations is literally to turn to Jesus and see him influencing my life on a day-to-day basis. And that seems to be lacking in some of what I hear.

Fr. Ashley: Well, of course, the fundamental principle of Christian morality is the imitation of Jesus. You are starting from the right point.

Question: Could you address the role of conscience in the case of a person who is involved in a second marriage, is convinced that the first marriage was invalid, but cannot obtain the necessary testimony for a marriage tribunal?

Fr. Ashley: You draw me a little far afield in the example you give. If, in conscience, the person believes the first marriage was invalid, then so far as he or she knows, the original marriage was not a real marriage and the present marriage may be valid. If in that case the person remained in that marriage, it would not be an issue of doing something intrinsically wrong. The problem of conscience is, however, what does this mean for the Christian community that someone is living in what appears to be an invalid marriage? The person *knows* it is not an invalid marriage, but it *appears* to be an invalid marriage. That provides some kind of scandal. It tends to break down the permanence of marriage within the Christian community. I do not need to settle here whether that is, in fact, sufficient to excuse the persons in a particular case. But these persons are not involved in something that is intrinsically wrong. Rather, this is a prudential question. The norm to avoid giving scandal is a nonabsolute norm, because occasions arise in which one cannot wholly avoid giving.

Question: In your system of beliefs, or your system of philosophy and theology, are you saying that life is an absolute value in all circumstances?

Fr. Ashley: I would say that innocent life is certainly an absolute value. That is why we cannot commit suicide. The problem, in view of Catholic tradition, is what about capital punishment? Previous theologians admitted that we could kill a criminal. That is under question now, however. It may be that this is like the slavery issue, that we have not been strict enough about this principle. Perhaps the value of life is such that it does not even permit capital punishment. That is debatable. Innocent life, though, is an absolute value. Even in war we do not have a right to kill the enemy directly. All we have a right to do is to try to prevent the enemy's aggressive action against us. But it cannot be the moral object, the intention of our act, to kill. This point is as old as Thomas Aquinas. The Church has never taught that you may directly kill somebody in war, but the Church has taught that you may stop aggression.

Question: Would you comment on the difference between the words *absolute value* and *inestimable value?*

Fr. Ashley: Perhaps inestimable might be a good word for an absolute value, because a person cannot measure one of these basic values against another basic value. You cannot say, for example, that a spiritual value can be measured over and against good health. We cannot simply sacrifice our bodily integrity to spiritual values. We must preserve both. In that sense they are inestimable, they are unmeasurable. We must try to preserve them all.

Question: Does inestimable mean that you keep on preserving life regardless of any other sort of factors?

Fr. Ashley: Well, I am not trying to address the question of the dying person and extraordinary and ordinary means of prolonging life, but we should not say that the dying person's life is something we can measure against some other good. That is not the right way to solve the problem. The right kind of question is, What can we do to preserve life? If nothing helpful can be done, then we are not required to do anything.

Question: And we preserve life because it has an absolute value, but not an inestimable value?

Fr. Ashley: No, it has both. An absolute value is inestimable. It is inestimable because you cannot measure it by weighing it against other values.

Question: Is there not a question about allowing a person to die and the use of ordinary and extraordinary means in the light of saying that life is an absolute value?

Fr. Ashley: Well, life *is* an absolute value as I see it. We try to do whatever we can for it. But the medical problem here is that there comes a point where we can do no more to preserve a life except keep a person in a coma or in pain and prolonged dying. Then we do not have the obligation to use our inadequate medical means. But, on the other hand, because human life is an absolute value, we have no right to take it. We cannot simply kill the suffering person. Proportionalism could lead to the conclusion that in some cases one would have a right to kill a person directly. If we are concerned about absolute moral norms, we would never be able to kill an innocent person, but we could be permitted to let that person die in certain circumstances.

Legal and Judicial Issues of Ethics Committees

Paul W. Armstrong

Mr. Armstrong, counsel for the Karen Quinlan family, reviews the way in which the New Jersey Supreme Court introduced the notion of an ethics committee in its decision about Karen Quinlan. He outlines several types of ethics committees and their appropriate function. He favors the use of such committees as more rapid and sensitive than judicial review but sees their function as recommending policy and giving counsel rather than making specific treatment decisions.

Our shared inquiry concerns the way in which the law, through its court and legislatures, views the notion of ethics committees. It is not necessary to catalog the cases and enactments that currently require or allow such groups but rather to share the human as well as the legally formal genesis and promise of this decisional process.

There was a time, not long ago, when we might have employed a number of hypothetical instances in order to underscore the notions implicit in the right of individuals to make fundamental treatment decisions while terminally ill. (Note that I have eschewed the so-called right to die; American law has not, does not, and, in all probability, will not recognize so broad a prerogative.) The necessity for hypothetical situations, however, has been obviated in that recent brief span of time in which Karen Ann Quinlan and Barney Clark have captured the interest and empathy of the world —a mere eight years.

Along with concerns for Miss Quinlan and Dr. Clark, the issue of the treatment of the terminally ill, competent and incompetent, the infant, the adult, the elderly, and the retarded has been the subject

Mr. Armstrong is Counsellor at Law, Bridgewater, NJ.

of considerable scrutiny. Nowhere else is this more plainly manifest than in the report *Deciding to Forego Life-Sustaining Treatment,* issued under the auspices of the President's Commission for the Study of Ethical Problems in Medicine and Biomedical and Behavioral Research.[1] This essay will attempt to sketch the history, promise, and problems of the so-called ethics committee.

The Notion of Ethics Committees and the Quinlan Case

The notion of an ethics committee received widespread attention as a result of its incorporation by the New Jersey Supreme Court in its landmark decision, *In the matter of Karen Ann Quinlan,* of March 31, 1976. A number of sister states, through their respective state supreme courts and legislatures, have done so as well, and many institutions have followed their example in forming their own deliberative mechanisms in the absence of a specific legal requirement to do so.

What has emerged from the public and private travail of *Quinlan* and its progeny are particular procedures that are premised on the constitutional right of privacy. They spring from a central concept that the individual may in certain circumstances refuse medical treatment, even if death is a likely result, and that, certain individuals may, in the best interests of incompetent persons, refuse treatment on their behalf. These principles have evolved from the situations of young and old alike and thus have broad application to the terminally ill of all ages.

The bishop of Paterson, NJ, Lawrence B. Casey, who at the time of *Quinlan* was dying of cancer, presaged the court's creation of the so-called ethics committee when he submitted the following call in the form of an amicus curiae brief before the New Jersey Supreme Court on behalf of all the Catholic bishops of New Jersey:

Medicine with its combination of advanced technology and professional ethics is both able and inclined to prolong biological life.

Law with its felt obligation to protect the life and freedom of the individual seeks to assure each person's right to live out his human life until its natural and inevitable conclusion.

45

Theology with its acknowledgment of man's dissatisfaction with biological life as the ultimate source of joy proclaims the individual's call to an endless sharing in a divine life beyond all corruptions. It also defends the sacredness of human life and defends it from all direct attacks.

These disciplines do not conflict with one another, but are necessarily conjoined in the application of their principles in a particular instance such as that of Karen Ann Quinlan. Each must in some way acknowledge the other without denying its own competence. The *civil law* is not expected to assert a belief in eternal life; nor, on the other hand, is it expected to ignore the right of the 1ndividual to profess it, and to form and pursue his conscience in accord with that belief.

Medical science is not authorized to direct!y cause natural death; nor, however, is it expected to prevent it when it is inevitable and all hope of a return to an even partial exercise of human life is irreparably lost.

Religion is not expected to define biological death; nor, on its part, is it expected to relinquish its responsibility to assist man in the formation and pursuit of a correct conscience as to the acceptance of natural death when science has confirmed its inevitability beyond any hope, other than that of preserving biological life in a merely vegetative state.

The common concern of the three disciplines as they focus on the situation of Karen Ann Quinlan is that of life and death. This fact demonstrates the need for theology, medicine, and law to develop an even greater interrelationship in an open, continuing, and growing dialogue on the profound issues arising from the biological revolution, a designation aptly applied to the age in which we live.[2]

What better way to foster such a dialog and at the same time obviate the need for juridical intervention than the diffusion of decision-making authority through an ethics committee?

The New Jersey Supreme Court, after vindicating Karen's constitutional right of decision through her surrogate father and guardian, responded as follows to whether continuing judicial involvement in this area was necessary:

There must be a way to free physicians, in the pursuit of their healing vocation, from possible contamination by self-interest or self-protection concerns which would inhibit their independent medical judgments for the well-being of their dying patients. We would hope that this opinion might be serviceable to some degree in ameliorating the professional problems under discussion.[3]

A technique aimed at the underlying difficulty (although in a somewhat broader context) is described by Karen Teel, MD, a pediatrician and a director of pediatric education, who writes in the *Baylor Law Review* under the title, "The Physician's Dilemma: A Doctor's View: What the Law Should Be." Dr. Teel recalls:

Physicians, by virtue of their responsibility for medical judgments, are, partly by choice and partly by default charged with the responsibility of making ethical judgments which we are sometimes ill-equipped to make. We are not always morally and legally authorized to make them. The physician is thereby assuming a civil and criminal liability that, as often as not, he does not even realize as a factor in his decision. There is little or no dialogue in this whole process. The physician assumes that his judgment is called for and, in good faith, he acts. Someone must, and it has been the physician who has assumed the responsibility and the risk.

I suggest that it would be more appropriate to provide a regular forum for more input and dialogue in individual situations and to allow the responsibility of these judgments to be shared. Many hospitals have established an ethics committee composed of physicians, social workers, attorneys, and theologians:.which serves to review the individual circumstances of ethical dilemmas and which has provided much in the way of assistance and safeguards for patients and their medical caretakers. Generally, the authority of these committees is primarily restricted to the hospital setting and their official status is more that of an advisory body than of an enforcing body.

The concept of an ethics committee which has this kind of organization and is readily accessible to those persons rendering medical care to patients would be, I think, the most promising direction for further study at this point.

[This would allow] some much needed dialogue regarding these issues and [force] the point of exploring all of the options for a particular patient. It diffuses the responsibility for making these judgments. Many physicians, in many circumstances, would welcome this sharing of responsibility. I believe that such an entity could lend itself well to an assumption of a legal status which would allow courses of action not now undertaken because of the concern for liability.[4]

The New Jersey Supreme Court wrote that the most appealing factor in the technique suggested by Dr. Teel seems to be the diffusion of professional responsibility for decisions, comparable in a way to the value of multijudge courts in finally resolving on appeal difficult questions of law. Moreover, such a system would protect the hospital as well as the physician in screening out, so to speak, a case that might be contaminated by less than worthy motivations of family or physician. In the real world and in relationship to the momentous decision contemplated, the value of additional views and diverse knowledge is apparent.

The court considered that applying to a court to confirm such decisions would generally be inappropriate, not only because that would be a gratuitous encroachment on the medical profession's field of competence, but because it would be impossibly cumbersome. Such a requirement is distinguishable from the judicial overview traditionally required in other matters, such as the adjudication and commitment of mental incompetents. This is not to say that in any case of an otherwise justiciable controversy access to the courts would be foreclosed; the court speaks rather of a general practice and procedure.

Although the deliberations and decisions that the court described would be professional, they should obviously include at some stage the feelings of the family of an incompetent relative. Decision making within health care, if it is considered as an expression of the physician's primary obligation, *primum non nocere,* should be controlled primarily within the patient-physician-family relationship.

If there could be created not necessarily this particular system of ethics committees but some reasonable counterpart, the court had no doubt that such decisions, thus determined to be in accordance with medical practice and prevailing standards, would be accepted by society and by the courts, at least in cases comparable to that of *Quinlan.*

The evidence in that case convinced the court that the focal point of the decision should be the prognosis of the reasonable possibility of a person's return to cognitive and sapient life, as distinguished from the forced continuance of that biological vegetative existence to which Karen Quinlan seemed doomed.

The court then set forth the following declaratory relief:

> Upon the concurrence of the guardian and family of Karen, should the responsible attending physicians conclude that there is no reasonable possibility of Karen's ever emerging from her present comatose condition to a cognitive, sapient state and that the life-support apparatus now being administered to Karen should be discontinued, they shall consult with the hospital "Ethics Committee" or like body of the institution in which Karen is then hospitalized. If that consultative body agrees that there is no reasonable possibility of Karen's ever emerging from her present comatose condition to a cognitive, sapient state, the present life-support system may be withdrawn and said action shall be without any civil or criminal liability therefore on the part of any participant, whether guardian, physician, hospital or others. We herewith specifically so hold.[5]

The Role and Functions of Ethics Committees

From this beginning, Professor Robert M. Veatch asserts that four general types of hospital committees have developed:

1. Committees to review the ethical and other values involved in individual patient care decisions

2. Committees to make larger ethical and policy decisions

3. Committees for counseling

4. Prognosis committees[6]

The President's commission has also found that the procedures that institutions have established, after *Quinlan,* to promote effective decision making for incapacitated individuals can serve a number of specific functions:

• They can review the case to confirm the responsible physician's diagnosis and prognosis of a patient's medical condition.

• They can provide a forum for discussion of broader social and ethical concerns raised by a particular case; such bodies may also have an educational role, especially in teaching all professional staff how to identify, frame, and resolve ethical problems.

• They can be a means for formulating policy and guidelines regarding such decisions.

• Finally, they can review decisions made by others (such as physicians and surrogates) about the treatment of specific patients or make such decisions themselves.[7]

In the main, such committees frequently perform all these tasks in their deliberations, regardless of the more narrow confines under which they were established.

Statistically, the report of the President's commission is not encouraging about the establishment of such committees throughout the country; the report states that "a national survey done for the Commission found that less than 1 percent of all hospitals—and just 4.3 percent of the hospitals with over 200 beds—have such committees."[8] I am happy to report that the Catholic Health Association (CHA) pointed out that a 1983 survey of Catholic hospitals showed that 41 percent of the respondents had established medical-moral committees.[9] The present volume, which studies the role and formation of ethics committees in Catholic health care, attests to the leadership role that Catholic institutions have assumed in exploring the ultimate efficacy of the ethics committee.

For scholars at CHA, the Pope John XXIII Medical-Moral Research and Education Center, the Kennedy Institute for Bioethics, the Hastings Center, and the President's commission, the first issue of concern is the ethics committee's appropriate role or function.

Perhaps the narrowest charter to be found is that of the so-called prognosis committee, whose task is limited to confirming the diagnosis and prognosis of a particular patient. Of necessity the committee must be confined to physicians and, more often than not, to specialists. Thus, the larger dialogs called for by *Quinlan* and the President's commission and CHA are patently unachievable in this form.

A second kind of committee, with perhaps the broadest mandate, would review the values in individual instances and make larger ethical and policy decisions. Such committees are concerned not only with the patient's condition, but also with the ramifications of the choices that the patient, family, physician, institutions, and society face. These committees would have members from many disciplines and thus be more able to recognize and reconcile the competing interests attendant upon many hard choices.

A third category of committee currently existing is that of the counseling committee established to provide to the patient and his or her family or to the health care provider or to both its counsel and advice about particular cases. These committees require specialists in the psychological and social sciences and in other areas as needed.

Right of Decision Making

An implicit and fundamental question for all these committees is whether the final decision in a particular case rests with the committee. Are ethics committees the actual decision makers, or do they merely consult and advise? The President's commission reports that fewer than 20 percent of the committees classified the making of final decisions about life-support as a stated purpose and slightly more than 30 percent classified this as an actual function.[10]

I think, along with the members of the President's commission, that regularly assigning to ethics committees the task of making decisions on life-sustaining treatment could undermine recognizing the obligations of those who should be principally responsible. The surrogates for an incapacitated person and the health care professionals should be the primary decision makers who, through the vehicle of an ethics committee, seek the keener insight of an interdisciplinary view in deciding on their course of action.

The tone of committees' inquiry should be one of fellow travelers wrestling with important decisions and not that of an adversary. The Anglo-Saxon premise that the truth will emerge from combat has no place in the sensitive convening of patient, family, physician, nurse, staff, and institution.

I have labored through this nation in the vineyard of its trial courts with these issues and can say candidly, from such experience, that often the illness itself presents less of a burden to all concerned than requiring the additional hardships—physical, financial, and psychological—of public juridical resolution of sacred and private family tragedies.

Several years ago, I was privileged to participate in a Hasting's Center conference, which was funded by the Ford Foundation, that analyzed the fledgling forms of ethics committees that had developed in New Jersey and Massachusetts after the *Quinlan* and *Saikewicz* decisions. Only a few months ago, and after years of hearings and study, the President's commission issued its lengthy report entitled *Deciding to Forego Life-Sustaining Treatment— Ethical, Medical, and Legal issues in Treatment Decisions.* Today we continue to face the same questions concerning the need, form, and function of ethics committees whose promise for our particular institutions seems boundless.

The President's commission, like the group at the Hastings Center, "believes that ethics committees and other institutional responses can be more rapid and sensitive than judicial review: They are closer to the treatment setting, their deliberations are informal and typically private (and are usually regarded by their participants as falling within the general rules of medical confidentiality), and they are able to reconvene easily or delegate decisions to a separate group of members."[11]

The commission further charges that, whatever the precise nature of the policies formulated, "institutions should recognize and evaluate the problems posed by the need to make decisions for incapacitated persons and should ensure that the decisions made promote their well-being."[12] To provide a basis for evaluating the different forms of decision making, it is especially important that institutions be explicit about the practices they adopt and that they report their successes and failures.

The Future: Refinement and Study

Two facts are apparent from this brief review of the important studies and cases concerning ethics committees. First, as far as the courts and legislatures are concerned, the verdict concerning the efficacy of the ethics committee as a proper vehicle for sharing medical decision making has yet to be reached. Second, the President's commission has issued an appeal to all involved to develop practices and procedures that will not only serve proper decision making but also provide the necessary data for a considered and scholarly analysis of ethics committees' growth, form, and function.

Let us issue a call to refine existing reporting procedures and to commission a comprehensive study to satisfy the felt need for serious inquiry into the workings of these various committees. I have seen in courts and legislatures throughout this country, and in Europe as well, that, historically, the burden of the ethical analysis of the dilemmas of modern science and medicine has fallen on the Catholic Church and its member institutions. This fact is heartening; it makes me proud of the special privilege of contributing these reflections and sharing in these important labors.

Notes

1. President's Commission for the Study of Ethical Problems in Medicine and Biomedical and Behavioral Research, *Deciding to Forego Life-Sustaining Treatment,* (Washington, DC: U.S. Government Printing Office, March, 1983).

2. Lawrence B. Casey, "A Statement on the Case of Karen Quinlan," *Catholic Mind,* (March 1976): 16-17.

3. *In the Matter of Karen Quinlan* 70 N.J. 10, cert. denied sub num., Garger V. New Jersey, 429 U.S. 922 (1976).

4. Karen Teel, "The Physician's Dilemma; A Doctor's View: What the Law Should Be." *Baylor Law Review* 76 (1975): 8-9.

5. Quinlan, 70 N. J. 55.

6. Robert M. Veatch, "What Is the Scope of Hospital Ethics Committees?" *Hospital Medical Staff* 6 (1977): 24-30.

7. President's Commission, pp. 160-161.

8. President's Commission, pp. 443-449.

9. Sr. Joan Kalchbrenner, RHSJ, Sr. Margaret John Kelly, DC and Rev. Donald McCarthy, "Ethics Committees and Ethicists in Catholic Hospitals," *Hospital Progress* 64 (September 1983): 47-51.

10. President's Commission, pp. 451.

11. President's Commission, pp. 168-169.

12. President's Commission, pp. 170.

Discussion After Mr. Armstrong's Lecture

Question: Would you mind looking at the *Quinlan* case a bit more for us? What caused the case to go to the courts in the first place? Second, what has happened to Karen? This may raise the question of the validity of prognostic decisions.

Mr. Armstrong: Let us answer the second question first, because I think it will be easier to respond to. At the time of trial, seven physicians from throughout the country testified concerning the probability that Karen would survive after the respirator had been removed. In the main, the testimony can be summarized as saying that she would not survive it. A number of physicians, however, advised that there was a real possibility that Karen could survive and survive for some time. Implicit in that question is something that I want to make clear: Karen is not medically unique. There are other individuals in that persistent vegetative state that have lived as long as and longer than Karen.

How could something like that have happened, and why could not the powers of persuasion have been applied that would have precluded the necessity for going to court in the first instance? The initial treating physicians had advised that Karen be removed from the respirator when it became apparent that the kind of care and treatment she was then receiving could offer no hope of cure or recovery. Karen was transferred from that hospital to a second hospital. It then become apparent to authorities at the second hospital that the treatment should not be continued. They broached the subject with the physician, who subsequently broached it with the Quinlan family, who finally decided that the respirator should be removed.

Meanwhile, that particular physician broached the subject with his mentor in New York City, who advised him of the kind of human crosscurrents that had developed and where he would be found in the context of those crosscurrents. This led to the inability to resolve this issue without going to court. As a matter of fact, the hospital had suggested that the case go to court so that it could be appointed guardian to make these kinds of decisions. We thought that would be inappropriate and tried to avoid it as best we could.

Question: In your experience, would so-called living wills perhaps conflict with ethics committees?

Mr. Armstrong: My starting point is that the constitutional right of privacy is something that should be held sacred. If you can draft a so-called living will, which does not in any way derogate from that higher standard of constitutional protection, but sets forth the proper vehicle so that individuals can exercise the constitutional right of privacy to make decisions on how they want to be treated when they are terminally ill, I am for it. The bill must allow for competing interests, e.g., the right to make that decision and, at the same time, the right to revoke it. Also, physicians need a lucid document in order to carry out a patient's wishes. If a uniform document is not required, physicians and attorneys would generally not want to interpret a living will but would allow the disease process to take its natural course before suspending treatment.

My general response is, if the living will bill can be drafted to be complementary to the constitutional right of privacy, and if it seems practically feasible, then it should be tried in order to preclude the necessity for going to court each and every time the issue arises.

Question: Ethics is a very difficult matter to define, and it seems to me that ethical decisions, as I know them, involve the input of many people besides ethicists and hospital administrators. But I do not know about extrapolating one extraordinary case to justify an ethics committee.

Mr. Armstrong: In America, which is a litigious society, we find ourselves at a crossroads. When a court is confronted with these questions, it can do one of two things procedurally. It can accept and hold as a matter of future procedure all questions arising from this particular technical innovation, or it can attempt to set up a system that would obviate the necessity for petitioning a court to resolve these hard choice questions.

The New Jersey Supreme Court adopted a philosophy, for the residents of the state of New Jersey, whereby it is inappropriate to mandate the necessity that cases like *Quinlan* continually come before the courts. What is a reasonable alternative that would meet the courts' responsibility to do justice and protect life, yet at the same time not overburden medicine or the patient and the patient's family? In searching out the literature, the court then found the suggestion of Dr. Karen Teel and decided that this would be an appropriate way of resolving those questions and, one hopes, of obviating the necessity to come to court.

Massachusetts arrived at a different conclusion in *Saikewicz,* for which it was severely criticized, and it has retreated posthaste from that position. The justices said that questions like this are so sacred and so fundamental that, as justices, they could not abrogate their responsibility to address these questions, although they have since retreated from this position. The genesis from *Quinlan,* since it was a case of first impression and the one that first looked to these issues, was the suggestion that the so-called ethics committee be adopted as a way of preserving physician, patient, and family autonomy while, at the same time, meeting the responsibility to protect life. That is the position today.

Question: Have we begun to change the ethics of and goals in medicine in the patient-physician relationship, the physician's view of medicine, society's view of medicine, and society's view of the patient?

Mr. Armstrong: I think that most of the Supreme Court justices and legislators realize that there is a danger of the breakdown of the primary community of family and patient. I think the main goal of everyone seriously laboring in this area is to try to protect the family as a unit. I think the problem is not so much that there is an adversary relationship between physicians and health care providers on the one hand, and the courts on the other hand. Rather, as science advances, its ramifications cause problems that the courts reach some 5 to 10 years after they have actually been created. I see more of an historical process with everybody trying to arrive at the same goal, that is, to re-protect what has worked for hundreds of years—that primacy of the physician-patient relationship.

Question: It seems to me that in the 33 years that I have been a physician I have seen two numbing things occurring in the care of patients in hospitals. One is the absolute unassailability of the American juridical system. No one dares question a lawyer; therefore, no one dares question defensive medicine. Lawyers are the absolute saviors and guardians of those most essential rights. That has brought a loss of trust. The second thing is the diminishing length of stay in the hospital. The great desirability to decrease the length of stay and defensive medicine are, I think, major problems.

Mr. Armstrong: Ethics committees are trying to prevent the necessity for recourse to court. The interposition of lawyers at the bedside and/or into the physician-patient relationship is a problem that has arisen because of technological growth and the way that America treats its citizens medically. Clearly, those involved in health care must recognize those problems and to try to set forth, in good faith, some way of resolving them.

Question: We have cases in which we have reluctantly put a patient on a respirator, and then the family has said, "Well, once you put him on, you cannot take him off." So we would have been better off not to put this patient on at all. Does that sound right?

Mr. Armstrong: We argue that situation as follows: If you had applied a modality of support, in this instance a respirator, and it had proved not to be of any curative value, offering no hope of cure or recovery to the patient, then we argue that *a fortiori,* with stronger reasoning, at least you tried it and proved that it did not work. Therefore, you are now on better grounds in removing it than if you had not tried it in the first place.

Question: We are looking at ever-decreasing amounts of health care resources in my country, Australia, and we are, consequently, being faced with the ethical problems of determining who should get those resources. Therefore, ethics committees will, of course, become important to us. How do we ensure that the patient and the physician in charge of that patient are represented on any ethics committee that is formed?

Mr. Armstrong: If we could find two elements that absolutely must be included in an ethics committee, exclusive of an historical context, they are the view of the patient and family and the view of the physician. No matter what else changes, these two ingredients must be included. In chartering the responsibilities and picking the members of the committee, those two goals should be primary.

Question: An article about two or three weeks ago in a popular publication spoke of a young, terminal patient who had been given "code blue" 52 times in one month. The patient had consistently refused consent for the procedure. It was the policy of the hospital, as it is the policy of many hospitals, that every patient be given the resuscitative procedure of "code blue" unless the physician signs an order to the contrary on the chart. Is this not assault and battery? Who is responsible? Does the hospital have the wrong policy? If the patient refuses "code blue" and the hospital says he or she must have it unless the physician signs the chart and the physician will not sign the chart, what are the legal implications?

Mr. Armstrong: The classic analysis of the circumstances in that case would hold that the "code blue" procedure is an assault and battery, since it was done against a competent patient's will. I would advise both the institution and his treating physician not to continue carrying out that procedure. In addition, the professional status of both the institution and the physician are jeopardized, since this situation could be construed as unprofessional conduct, which could lead to the forfeiture of both sets of licenses. The real practical problem is that in the context of a civil suit there will be a jury trial. The prosecutor will charge that the physician repeatedly assaulted the patient and precluded the dying process from running its natural course, to the detriment, pain, and suffering of the patient as well as his family. The defense for the physician will cite the axiom, *primum non nocere,* that the first mandate is to do no harm, to protect life, not to end it, and to follow prevailing medical standards. It is conceivable that a jury in a large metropolitan area could come back with $1 million or $1.5 million damages assessed against the physician and the institution. It is also conceivable that the jury could come back with nothing; the jury might determine that the physician was following the mandates of the profession. So, in a way, the question is not answered by a lawsuit. It is answered by raising the issue and making both physicians and institutions sensitive to the fact that depersonalization is very real and easy to hide in a large hospital.

Question: The Catholic Church should be in a position of leadership, but where do we go from here?

Mr. Armstrong: Wherever I go in the country, and questions such as this arise, the first individuals who are called to help resolve them, whether it is in the legislature or in the courts, are the local bishop, the Chancery office staff, and the ethicist of that particular diocese. Historically, this responsibility has devolved upon Catholics. We must now meet this responsibility so as not to be caught later in a situation like that of the abortion controversy.

Corporate Conscience: Governance and Management
Sr. Miriam Therese Larkin, CSJ

Sr. Larkin describes the notion of corporate conscience because ethics committees are called to reflect the moral principles of a Catholic corporate conscience in their work. She points out that general moral principles need practical implementation in the specific setting of a health care institution. While the sponsoring group, the board, and the administrative team all undertake this task to some degree, the ethics committee can offer invaluable assistance.

In this chapter I will examine the concept of corporate conscience, dividing my remarks into five areas: (1) general comments about the concept of corporate conscience; (2) what conscience is and how it functions; (3) identifying the self as Catholic through one's conscience; (4) applying conscience to a health care facility; and (5) some problems in applying conscience. Although the five areas do tend to overlap, the division is useful for purposes of discussion.

Corporate Conscience

The notion of corporate conscience is, like the notion of a corporate person, a legal fiction. In order to ascribe legal responsibility to corporations, the law created the fictitious corporate person with legal agency. It can be sued or can sue; acquire and alienate property; unite with other persons to make contracts, and prosper or go bankrupt. Because we attribute legal and moral responsibility to corporations, we therefore also attribute to them a conscience.[1]

In other words, we may speak of corporate conscience only analogously with personal conscience. We cannot strictly apply to it all that holds true for the concept of personal conscience.

Sr. Larkin, formerly professor of philosophy at Mount St. Mary's College, Los Angeles, is general superior, Sisters of St. Joseph of Carondelet, St. Louis, MO.

Nevertheless, the concept of corporate conscience is essential and must be used insofar as corporations have moral and legal responsibility and as social sin is a reality.

What Conscience Is and How It Functions

A look at the concept of personal conscience allows us to draw from it some applications for the concept of corporate conscience. Personal conscience is a person's concrete judgment of his or her own immediate action; it is the final norm by which the action must be guided. Conscience is a dictate of the practical intellect or reason by which a person judges, by speculation and examination, whether a particular act is good and should be performed or evil and should be avoided. It is, in short, the application of knowledge to a specific action. What needs to be emphasized here is that the action of conscience has to do with one's own actions, not the actions of others. For instance, if I judge others' actions as right or wrong, that is not a judgment of my conscience. Although the judgment draws on my perception of values, it is not a judgment of conscience. The action of conscience concerns the actions that I have performed or am about to perform.[2]

This function of conscience in judging the rightness and wrongness of action implies two things. First, the person with a conscience has a general sense of value, an awareness of personal responsibility characteristic of human beings; she is accountable and has the capacity for self-direction. Second, it implies that the person has a specific perception of values—concrete individual values—that emerge in the external processes of reflection, discussion, and analysis in which persons and corporations engage. It is at this level of searching that a person may differ with others and disagree.[3]

If we apply this idea to corporations, we may say that the corporation exercises its conscience insofar as the corporation makes concrete judgments about what should be done or avoided in actions for which it is responsible. This presumes that the corporation has a general sense of value, is aware of personal responsibility, is accountable, has the capacity for self-direction, and engages in an ongoing process of reflection, discussion, and analysis to develop its specific perception of values, i.e., its concrete individual values.

Conscience and Self-Identification as Catholic

How does an institution identify itself as Catholic through its conscience? To have a conscience presumes that one has a general sense of value, an awareness of responsibility, and the capacity for self-direction. Here the point of being a Catholic institution is significant. Conscience requires that we understand who we are and are faithful to it. A Catholic is one committed to carrying out Jesus' mission in his or her specific area of life and action. The Catholic conscience is thus one that understands Jesus' mission and is faithful to it; i.e., one who attends to what is to be done or avoided in carrying out Jesus' mission in any endeavor. It is not simply a matter of doing good and avoiding evil, of carrying out moral principles but also of responding to the higher imperative of one's commitment—fidelity to the mission of Jesus—that, I believe, takes us beyond questions of doing good or avoiding evil.

Second, to have a conscience presumes that one has a specific perception of concrete individual values and also that one engages in an ongoing process of reflection, discussion, and analysis. One's values are identified and emerge in this ongoing process. In this process of reflection, a personal or corporate conscience that is Catholic recognizes the Church as a teacher of moral values and listens to the Church, not because there is no possibility that the Church can err, but because the Holy Spirit stands with the Church, not protecting it in all things from error, but guiding it. Therefore, to listen to the Church is the reasonable and prudent thing to do.

The process of reflection in which Catholics engage is necessary not only for determining what is right and wrong but also for helping the Church. The "Decree on Divine Revelation" tells us that tradition develops in the Church in two ways: first, by the study and contemplation of all believers; second, by the teachings of the bishops.[4] The reflection in which a Catholic engages is part of assisting in the development of Church tradition.

Here I want to emphasize that it is not sufficient to listen to the Church's moral teachings. It is also required that one continually reflect on Jesus' mission as expressed in the Gospels, that one continually reflect on the goals of that mission and the manner in which it is carried out. The Church has not spoken explicitly on every practical moral implication of the Gospel. For example, the

Church has not spoken out on the obligation of giving persons information about their own health in language that they can understand, yet this is a requirement of human dignity, one of the basic Christian principles. In other words, if we only look at what the Church specifically tells us we must do, our reflection is incomplete. Let us suppose that the Church had no ethical or moral teachings, that it had never made a public statement on any ethical implication of the Gospel. Given the fact that a person or institution identifies itself as committed to Jesus' mission, it would be ethically obligated to reflect on the nature of that mission and its implications for those who identify with or participate in it.

Finally, conscience as a concrete judgment about one's own action is Catholic in that it applies the Church's insight and guidance to its judgments about what should be done or avoided. This does not mean that the answers to life's questions and the decisions about the rightness or wrongness of one's actions are simply dictated by agents outside ourselves. Moral agents are characterized by knowledge and freedom; they must make their own decisions and think through the reasons for a given decision in the light of their motives and principles and the circumstances of the situation. This is the prudential judgment that Abp. Pilarczyk discussed earlier.

Applying Conscience to a Health Care Facility

A health care facility (or any corporation) has implicit in its structure some factors that make it difficult to apply the concept of person or conscience to it. The functioning of conscience in an individual requires a level of maturity that is the result of years of development. It requires a unity in the self whereby the self deliberates and acts.[5]

By its nature, a corporation does not have that unity of "self" organically but only artificially, since in a corporation responsibility and decision making are divided. The agent who is ultimately responsible is often not the one who makes the concrete decisions. The sponsoring group that may own the institution creates decision making boards to act on its behalf with certain reservations. The sponsoring group or congregation must clearly define the facility's philosophy, mission, and role, but the board of trustees makes many of the decisions that give expression to the institution's philosophy, mission, and role. In addition, management and employees make even more specific decisions about day-to-day functioning that give concrete expression to the facility's philosophy and mission.[6]

All this implies that the unity necessary for the corporate conscience's proper functioning is something that must be worked for very deliberately. True, the sponsoring group must clearly define and promulgate its own philosophy and mission to the board and must have adequate means for calling for accountability. The same is true of the board of trustees: It must clearly understand the institution's philosophy and mission and be able to promulgate it. It too should have mechanisms for calling for accountability from management.[7]

The division and delegation of a health care facility's rights and responsibilities require unity in the vision and goals of the sponsoring group, the board, and all the personnel who make decisions. Surely this requires constant reflection on the mission and goals of the institution. Who engages in this ongoing process of reflection? It is not sufficient that any one of the groups—sponsoring group, board, management, employees—engage in the process by itself. The corporation's values are identified by the sponsoring group but they are expressed in concrete decisions by the board, management, and employees. In the end, the sponsoring group is ultimately responsible for striving for this responsibility, i.e., for seeing that the institution's conscience functions at the most concrete level of action. How can the sponsoring group provide for this? Ethics committees geared to education and action and not simply to responding to crises are one answer, but perhaps only a part of the answer.[8] Too often ethics committees deal only with medical-moral problems, yet ethics in a health care institution applies to much more than medical or patient care decisions.[9]

Some Problems In Applying Corporate Conscience

Finally, there are some problems inherent in the concept of corporate conscience. These afflict personal conscience also but become more serious in corporate conscience, where responsibility and decision making are often divided. In making decisions we often find ourselves in situations in which there is a conflict of values, principles, or rights. In those situations we must decide which right, value, or principle is primary. It is clear that the Church does not provide a hierarchy of values or principles that enables us to always choose the correct value or principle. We must do our own thinking in such cases, just as the Church has had to do its own thinking and has developed its thoughts on such issues as conscientious objection, pacifism, just war, and nuclear war. In making decisions in which there is a conflict of values, we may override a value that we believe is important. How do we know, in such cases, that the value or principle still is important to us? One way to test ourselves is to ask whether we are reluctant at having given second place to the value or principle in question. If we are, the value or principle is still important to us.[10] But how does a corporation experience reluctance or regret when responsibility and decision making are divided? Those who are ultimately responsible may regret having to make a decision that gives second place to an important principle, but those who carry out the concrete decision may be quite content with it. Again, this brings us to the problem of unity in the corporate self. There is an accepted principle in moral theology that one should not impose on conscience a burden that is too great for that conscience to bear. What is too great a burden differs from one person to another. Are there burdens that are too great for corporations to bear? What is relevant to resolving the question?

Other problems for corporate conscience are analogous to the problems that individuals experience in exercising personal conscience. One may have insufficient knowledge to make a conscientious decision. Who or what is responsible for that insufficiency? Or, there may be insufficient reflection. Americans are constantly bombarded by immediate concerns; as a result, reflection on long-range consequences or deeper values is sometimes difficult if not impossible. Moral blind spots may also afflict us personally or corporately. Even the Church has experienced her own moral blind spots in the course of history. Persons and corporations experience the need to be right, to be relevant, to be considered valuable, to enjoy approval, and to grow stronger or more powerful. All these drives may blind one to questions that must be asked and answered if one is to live authentically and morally.

Finally, the fear of death or disintegration may blind one to the questions that must be asked or to the perception of a greater good that must be done. Even corporations must consider the possibility that death must occur so that new life may grow.

In the matter of corporate conscience, there are more questions than answers at present. For a corporation to identify itself as Catholic is a serious matter that needs much more thought than has been given to it. As Abp. Pilarczyk said, quoting Thomas Hardy, "much is there waits you we have missed, much, much lays outside our ken."

Notes

1. Edward Stevens, *Business Ethics* (New York: Paulist Press, 1979), pp. 133-135.

2. Thomas Aquinas, *Summa Theologica,* I, q. 79, art. 13 (New York, Benziger Brothers, 1947). See also Timothy E. O'Connell, *Principles for a Catholic Morality* (New York: The Seabury Press, 1978), pp. 88-93.

3. O'Connell identifies these two implications of conscience as the first two functions of conscience, the act of judging being the third function. Even if one identifies the act of judging as the only function of conscience, the other two functions may be implied from that act.

4. A. Flannery, ed, "Dogmatic Constitution on Divine Revelation," art. 8, *Vatican Council II: The Conciliar and Post Conciliar Documents* (Collegeville, MN: The Liturgical Press, 1975), p. 754. "The Tradition that comes from the apostles makes progress in the Church, with the help of the Holy Spirit. There is a growth in insight into the realities and words that are being passed on. This comes about in various ways. It comes through the contemplation and study of believers who ponder these things in their hearts (cf. Lk 2:19 and 51). It comes from the intimate sense of spiritual realities which they experience. And it comes from the preaching of those who have received, along with their right of succession in the episcopate, the sure charism of truth. Thus, as the centuries go by, the Church is always advancing towards the plenitude of divine truth, until eventually the words of God are fulfilled in her."

5. John W. Glaser, "Conscience and Superego: A Key Distinction," in C. Ellis Nelson, ed, *Conscience: Theological and Psychological Perspectives* (New York: Newman Press, 1973), pp. 167-188.

6. Sr. Mary Maurita Sengelaub, RSM, "Governance, Sponsorship, Management: What is the Trustee's Role?" *Hospital Progress,* 63(July 1982): 75.

7. Sengelaub, p. 75.

8. See Sr. Diana Bader, OP, "Medical-Moral Committee: Guarding Values in an Ambivalent Society," *Hospital Progress,* 63(Dec. 1982): 80-83; Sr. Joan Kalchbrenner, RHSJ, Sr. Margaret John Kelly, DC, and Rev. Donald C. McCarthy, "Ethics Committees and Ethicists in Catholic Hospitals," *Hospital Progress,* 64(Sept. 1983): 47-51; Edward Lisson, SJ, "Active Medical Morals Committee: Valuable Resource for Health Care,: *Hospital Progress,* 63(Oct. 1982): 36-37, 68.

9. *Evaluative Criteria for Catholic Health Care Facilities* (St. Louis: The Catholic Health Care Association of the United States, 1980). The structure of this working document is based on the view that ethics in health care institutions is much more than a matter of medical practice or patient care issues.

10. I am indebted for this insight to Bernard Williams in his essay in Stuart Hampshire, ed, *Public and Private Morality* (Cambridge: Cambridge University Press, 1978).

Corporate Conscience: Governance and Management

Sr. Mary Roch Rocklage, RSM

Speaking from a very practical point of view, Sr. Rocklage envisions the exciting impact that effective ethics committees can have within a health care institution. She describes how ethics committees can undertake serious reflection about the ethical significance of the entire function of a health care facility, both medical and economic. She describes the educational mission which grows out of this experiential process and calls for the realization of a shared ethical vision.

It is only through a process of thoughtful reflection that we in the Catholic health care apostolate shall begin to realize and implement the potential of ethics committees. Indeed, careful attention to the nature and functions will not only renew our understanding of health care, it may even reform the Catholic health care ministry. Incorporating a process of ethical reflection helps address a nagging concern of some members of the sponsoring religious communities and others, who, although not members of religious communities, have given their lives to Catholic health ministry: "Why stay in the institutions? They are not relevant; they are big businesses. They do not effect significant change, so we should get out of them." Although this concern is raised less frequently now, it still comes up periodically. "Why should a religious community sponsor what seems to be nothing other than large businesses?" I contend that, if we really begin to implement a process of ethical reflection in our health care institutions and allow this process to inform our decisions, we will be using our corporate structures very effectively. Perhaps our corporate structures are not as alive and effective as they could be if we were to permeate them with the values we hold dear. Such a permeation might well transform what appears to be simply a big business into a vehicle for changing the system. I see ethics committees as having a tremendous potential for influencing our governance and management groups. If we implement this type of

Sr. Rocklage is Provincial Administrator, Sisters of Mercy, St. Louis Province, St. Louis, MO.

process within our system, we will strategically and very markedly affect the process of decision making. Most notably, we will affect the *quality* of the decisions made.

Our decisions cannot be made in isolation, dicated solely by business concerns, i.e., what is efficient and expedient. By bringing into play other dimensions and values through ethical reflection, we would affect the decision process itself. Our institutions would change, and our relationships would be different.

Definitions and Value Systems

Let me give a few definitions before continuing to develop my approach to ethics committees in relation to governance and management issues. *Governance* refers to the board of trustees of a corporation, while *management* refers to those responsible for an institution's day-to-day operations. Sr. Miriam defined *corporate conscience* well. It is corporate awareness put into effect so that we consciously know what we are doing when we make a broad policy that will be applied in formulating a specific decision. She said that specific decisions are not ordinarily made at the corporate level, but the bases or the criteria—the standards that will affect those decisions—must be reflected at the corporate level before the structures for individual decisions are established.

I have adopted a definition of ethics that is described in the booklet, *Ethics in Corporate Policy Process: An Introduction* published by the Center of Ethics and Social Policy at Berkeley. It states that "ethics is reflection on the moral meaning of action. Ethics does not offer a single absolute right way of behavior. Rather, it assists us to see more clearly and understand with greater precision what we probably are pretty much aware of already but dimly and inadequately."

Ethics is a process. It is not an answer. In this context, it is not a specific right or a wrong. When we talk about an ethics committee and its implications for the corporate conscience as well as for governance and management, we are speaking about a broad-based committee of men and women from various disciplines, whose charge is broader than a medical-moral committee or a committee that reviews research within the institution. It is a core of persons with diverse gifts and interests brought together to reflect on the multifacetedness of the many decisions to be made in the health care apostolate and the policies to be formulated.

If such a process is initiated at the corporate level as well as within individual hospitals and multi-institutional systems, we shall reform our institutions. This reflective process will permeate the entire enterprise. All decisions, not just medical-moral ones, will be viewed within the context of ethical reflection. The ethics committee functioning will be as effective and as powerful as we allow it to be by giving it status and making it important from the corporate level down.

Scope of Ethics Committees

I venture to say that we all have devised standards within our system or institution to measure financial viability. What is the rate of return? What is the policy on how finances will be organized, and how are the bottom line figures reached? How many of you have similar standards for pastoral ministry, i.e., not just pastoral care and visitation of patients but employee relations, business relations, the broad concept of pastoral ministry? Those are the standard measures of excellence that an ethics committee should pursue. With this broad-based challenge we begin to reflect on current and future issues.

Let me briefly suggest another way of approaching the topic of "Governance and Management: Implications of Corporate Conscience for Ethics Committees." Let us turn the title around to read: "The Ethics Committee and Its Implications for the Corporate Conscience: Governance and Management." Sr. Miriam described the first charge to the sponsoring group at the corporate level as articulating the value system. Without an articulated value system at a given institution, at the provincial or multi-institutional level, no ethics committee—or any other group, for that matter—will be able to function, because it will be operating in a vacuum. On the other hand, it is the institutional ethics committee that constitutes the very group of people who can help the volunteer and the employee to articulate and implement the value system.

Once the value system has been carefully articulated in a mission and philosophy statement, the ethics committee can use it as one part of its discussion of a particular issue. This ensures that the discussion takes into account various essential factors, e.g., the sponsoring community's charism and values, Church teachings, Gospel values, implications for the local Church. The committee considers the claims of the larger community, the insights of medical science, and the best interests of the institution(s) against the articulated mission and then formulates policy. We must also look at our vested interests.

The effectiveness of the ethics committee will depend on where it is placed within the institution and the relative weight it is accorded. There are several ways to do this. Not every institution has the wherewithal to have a broad-based ethics committee. If this is not possible, there are ways to regionalize an ethics committee at the provincial or system level to bring together the people necessary for a committee. An interdisciplinary group at the system level could reflect on a given issue and then develop a policy. Sweeping rules are not the goal; rather, the aim is to provide broad-based policies that will help our institutions reach informed decisions in particular cases. Ethics committees will not have answers to questions before they are raised. I see them as giving broad guidelines developed without undue haste and stripped of vested local interests.

The same thing can happen in the local institution, where the board of trustees for the corporation can appoint an ethics committee that will report directly to it. Such a group would ideally address current and anticipated issues.

Role of the Ethics Committee: Various Forms

The institutional ethics committee might serve an *anticipatory function,* addressing questions such as, "What are the issues that will arise regarding employees, medical staff, the local civic community, the question of competition, or medical-moral problems? What do we see on the horizon, given today's society?" On the basis of these questions and the perspectives they generate, the committee would draw up its agenda. It would take the time to reflect upon these questions, so that it did not make decisions based solely on efficiency and economy. Institutional policies—the rules, regulations, procedures, and criteria—must be examined annually so that we can go back from our lived experience and ask, "Have things changed? Do we need more change? Can we help further develop Church teaching and practice?

In addition to this anticipatory function, ethics committees can also serve an *educational function* in at least two ways. First, specific programs can be offered in individual institutions or throughout a system on difficult issues. In this way trustees and managers can acquaint persons with their policies and, at the same time, elicit their advice and opinions. Second, the ethics committee can carry out its educational function by showing the institution that very few black and white issues exist. Most of them are gray. Such an awareness takes time to cultivate; eventually, though, department heads and the committee will be able to engage in dialogue, seeking the best way to approach a variety of issues.

The ethics committee should not be charged with making final decisions but should rather be advising. Its role would not be to judge but to help, i.e., to reflect on a given decision or how to reach a decision about a given issue, knowing that the board of trustees is ultimately responsible for policy.

Scope of Committee

In addition to medical-moral issues, ethics committees can deal with other ethical questions. One significant area that an ethics committee might fruitfully address is the area of finances today in connection with caring for the indigent. Questions arising now are, "Do we ever say no? Is there going to be a time when we can say, 'We can do no more for the poor'?" How is this issue of caring for the indigent connected with the question of policies of those who sponsor or have physician office buildings? Can they refuse the poor? That may be an individual physician's decision, but what does that say about *us*? Do we have a responsibility to investigate such policies and try to effect a change or are our hands tied? Should we ask ourselves some serious questions in this regard?

The area of personnel relations presents another set of issues. What about basic compensation? When several hospitals come together to identify the values that they hold in light of the Gospel, the sponsoring community's particular charism, and Church teachings with regard to the person's basic dignity, they must ask some questions: What are our policies regarding basic minimum compensation? How about health care benefits, life insurance, retirement benefits? What are the basic benefits for our employees to which they have a right, and how much choice do we give them? What do we say to the young nurse who says, " I am 22 years old, and I would rather not put so much into retirement at this point." Can we give her a choice? Should we have flexible compensation programs?

Another issue for committee consideration—unions—is one which can be divisive. The question of unions, however, touches on the Church's teaching that individuals have a right to share in the power and authority of decisions that affect them. We must ask ourselves how we let our employees share in the power and in the authority of our institutions? Do our methods reflect our values?

Conclusions

Finally, committees can assist governance and management in the relentless search for truth which is our duty. Our relentless search for truth, our being faithful members of the Church and living out what we say we are, all give lived expression to our Christianity, our Catholicism, but it also makes our actions influential and relevant for today.

I envision our health care institutions not just centered on healing, but touching all levels and structures of society. If administration and governance will enter into the asceticism and discipline of planning and thinking ahead of time, we will become centers of peace and justice for the people whom we serve, those who serve with us, and for society and the Church at large. Some time ago, I heard someone ask, "How many of us ever thought of including categories like theologian, philosopher, or ethicist when discussing the makeup of our boards of trustees? We only think of businesspeople, lawyers, bankers. Why not the others?" Perhaps the arena where things move swiftly is not the best place for that kind of "heady talent. We would never get the work done, some might say. But if we believe in our mission, then we must set up the time for it. We need the right information—not just facts, but a genuine statement of values—to make the right decisions.

Discussion after the Lectures of Sr. Miriam Therese and Sr. Mary Roch

Question: I was thinking about the comment that Sr. Miriam Therese made about how much we do for the poor. A Scripture verse came to my mind, where Jesus says, "Those who want to save their life are going to lose it and if you are willing to lose your life for my sake then you'll save it." The question I would like to ask is, "Is it possible for corporations to be willing to lose their life?" How does that happen?

Sr. Miriam Therese: I think it is. One of the difficulties of dealing with that question in our society is that so much health care is available and the health care that is available is such high-technology health care. That is one of the reasons why it becomes difficult to serve the poor. I wonder if we have thought of all the possibilities, all the alternatives in serving the poor. Maybe we must die in one way to live in another way, which is what we all do in dying anyway.

Question: Sometimes in our employee orientation programs the extent of talking about the philosophy of our institutions is merely to say we are Catholic. Orientation is a good time to tell employees who we are and what we stand for. This orientation should not be limited to the executive staff. Our patients are going to be cared for in light of the Gospel, I believe, by all employees. I really believe that those of us who work with employees who give patient care can also set that example. Our hospital in the past years has made drastic changes in letting the people of our community know that we are Catholic. It is very hard sometimes to stand by those commitments, but it can be done.

Sr. Mary Roch: I agree strongly with you about the initial orientation, and I also believe that every one of our institutions should establish a program that allows us to vocalize our values. One of the things that should stand out about our hospitals is the lived reality that the person is in the image of God, and so our facilities reflect that. How we as staff deal with one another must also reflect that.

I once wrote a paper on the theme that we are so busy seeing Jesus in our patients we wipe our feet on our employees. We forget that they are the ones who minister with and for us, and so we must touch them and enliven them.

Sr. Miriam Therese: I could not agree with you more. I think as Catholics we sometimes tend to be very superficial about our commitment. It goes back to a kind of legalism from our past. When the Church speaks loudly and clearly on certain things, we think that if we are in accord with those, we have done everything we have to do. I do not think that's the case. We can tend very easily to think that if we follow Church teaching on abortion, sterilization, contraception, and life supports, we have done everything we need to do. That is why we have become so complacent.

We have heard that Harvard Medical School is interested in what we have to offer in terms of ethics committees. I want to tell you, though, what has been occurring at Harvard Medical School for years. Physicians have what they call "ethical rounds," where physicians come voluntarily and present cases somewhat anonymously. People are invited to the discussions, and the goal is to try to understand how to treat persons with dignity. Are we doing that in our Catholic institutions?

Question: We are involved in legislation to help the poor. But if a physician thinks that the state monies are not good enough, then we are out of business, too, no matter how much good will we have. We also have a parish Church owning a large professional building, lending their facility to people who refer or do abortions.

Sr. Mary Roch: If you could start at the very beginning, when you actually begin to have an office building on your premises that is identified with you, you can spell out within your lease as clearly as possible the ethical principles that your tenants must uphold. When that has not been done and the question is raised, you must sit down with the given physicians and try to get them to see how inconsistent referring for abortions is with the values you hold. Show them that when they are on your premises, they are identified with you.

Also, I feel sad when we do not find it a scandal when a physician refuses to take Medicaid patients. I think one of our greatest scandals down the road will be raised by how we have handled the poor. This is not our sole responsibility, certainly they aren't all ours to care for. It is a joint responsibility. There is a great scandal, if when there is more than one Catholic hospital in a given city, no one works together on meeting the needs of the poor.

Question: Ethics committees can be a resource not only, of course, for nursing students and the faculty but for everyone in the hospital community. Many former graduates feel they have nowhere else to turn in regard to problems dealing with the ethics of health care. It seems to me that if a Catholic hospital is bearing witness to its mission, it will have those resources within its own institution. I see an ethics committee as being the resource committee and also a comforting and helping committee.

Sr. Miriam Therese: I think your point is very good, and you also reminded me that many of us sponsor not only health care institutions, but health care institutions that have nursing schools or premed programs. What is the sponsoring congregations' responsibility with respect to the ethical component in these programs? This question needs serious reflection also.

Part Three
Contemporary Response: Formation and Function of Ethics Committees

Committee Formation and Function*

Experience has shown that careful preliminary planning will facilitate the development, as well as the effectiveness, of an ethics committee. Such preparation should focus on objectives, delineate accountabilities, and psychologically prepare the overall community in which the committee will function. Responses to the following key questions dictate how a committee will be formed and will subsequently function:

1. What are the principles and guidelines that will influence committee formation and functioning?

2. What is the scope of activity that will be referred to the committee?

Principles and guidelines. In responding to the first question, the preliminary planners will wish to identify principles and orientation that will provide overall consistent direction to the committee (what has previously been referred to as the corporate conscience), independent of the member's personal beliefs, experiences, and expertise. These encompass religious and secular principles and are depicted below. In regard to Church affiliation, convenors of committees must consider the bishop's role as teacher, the sponsoring group's stewardship accountabilities, and the place of the *Ethical and Religious Directives for Catholic Health Facilities.* Other chapters of this book have dealt with these sources in detail.

In addition to church guidance, legislative and judicial decisions that will affect the committee's work should also be identified. Persons considering forming a committee should know federal and state legislation on the necessity for and liability of such committees as well as the articulated provisions for an institution to follow its corporate conscience. They should also be aware of any case law relevant to the actions of their committees. Furthermore, some basic legal principles give direction in the development and activities of ethics committees:

---

*This chapter synthesizes the experiences of the panelists (identified in the preface) and the observations of the participants in the workshop.

- Patients have the right to make decisions about their care.

- The health care facility is responsible (liable) in a general way for the quality of care being rendered in it. This responsibility rests ultimately with the facility's governing board, which must make sure that sufficient policies and procedures are in place to ensure appropriate patient care.

- Patients' privacy rights must be respected. Because the physician-patient relationship is privileged and confidential, persons not directly involved in the patient's care must have the patient's permission to become privy to information that is identifiable as relating to the patient. (A consent form at the time of admission can provide for this.)

- Unless the physician is discharged from the patient's case or preempted by court order, specific treatment decisions remain the physician's responsibility. This implies informed consent by the patient for all treatment.

- Records of ethics committee activities can be discoverable and admissible in litigation and should be maintained with accuracy and fairness. (Recent leglislation in Louisiana now protects all hospital committee activity while other states have proposals regarding confidentiality and immunity.)

The diagram on the next page depicts the relationship of an ethics committee to its sources of formation and information.

Scope of the committee. In responding to the second question, planners will want to review the existing committee structure as well as the expertise available. Currently there are two approaches to the scope of issues addressed by ethics committees. The first, more comprehensive approach is based on the conviction that human rights provide the focus and thus the committee should concern itself with the whole sphere of human behavior issues such as clinical practice, management of investments, labor relations, and a variety of other social justice issues. The second, more specialized approach limits its attention to clinical or patient and resident care issues.

Source and Reference for Ethics Committee

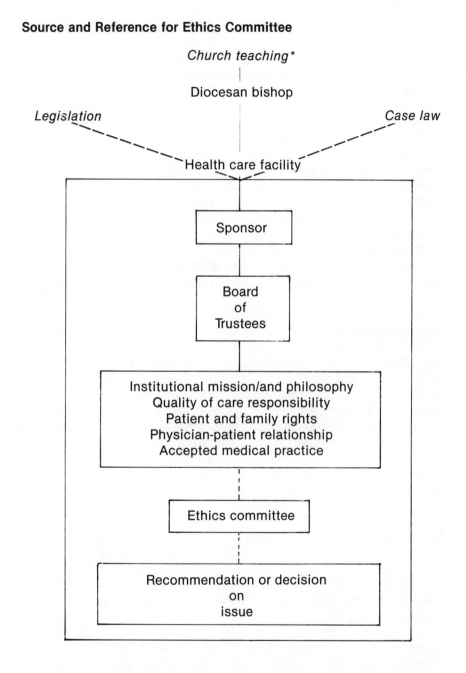

Church teaching*

Diocesan bishop

Legislation   *Case law*

Health care facility

Sponsor

Board
of
Trustees

Institutional mission/and philosophy
Quality of care responsibility
Patient and family rights
Physician-patient relationship
Accepted medical practice

Ethics committee

Recommendation or decision
on
issue

*Nondenominational institutions will want to identify certain key values
and principles to serve as a core of guidance for the committee.

The first type of committee is more appropriately designated as an ethics committee, while the second is, strictly speaking, a medical ethics or a bioethics committee. When either of these committees makes use of Christian revelation as well as human reason for its moral guidance, it is more appropriately called a Christian ethics committee or a Christian medical ethics or Christian bioethics committee. The term *medical-moral* committee as used in Catholic health facilities usually refers to a Christian medical ethics committee that relies ultimately on principles of Catholic moral theology and magisterial teaching of the Church for its moral guidance. (The glossary in the back of this book offers distinct definitions for ethics and Christian ethics; it describes medical-moral committees without adverting to the fact that in Catholic institutions they normally derive moral guidance specifically from Catholic theology and Church teaching. For convenience, in subsequent discussion, references will be made to an ethics committee without differentiating the scope.)

The advantage of the ethics committee that uses the more comprehensive approach is that it underscores the centrality of the person and unifies all the ethical reflection and decision making within a diocese, system, or institution. The obvious disadvantage is that it tends to be unmanageable both in scope of activity and in ensuring the appropriate range of competence in its members. The advantage of the medical ethics committee is that it has a specific focus and concentrates on the major purpose and competence of the health care facility. Of course, the disadvantage is that it divorces medical issues from the broader range of human ethical issues.

Next, the guiding principles and scope of the committee should be succinctly summarized and prepared for the committee members-to-be. Persons concerned with the formation of the committee must then turn to the substantive questions of purpose and function, membership and accountability, and operational guidelines. The following three sections of this chapter discuss these various topics as they relate to ethics committees at the (1) institutional, (2) diocesan, and (3) system level. In addition, questions and observations made by participants and panelists in the workshop are summarized, and a model for an institutional committee is presented.

Institutional Committees

Purpose and function. Generally speaking, institutional committees, whether they are general ethics or medical ethics committees, are developed for at least some of the following purposes:

1. Policy review

2. Policy recommending

3. Policy making

4. Case advisory

5. Case decision making

6. Retrospective case review

7. Educational programming

Traditionally within Catholic facilities, the two primary purposes appear to be policy recommending and educational programming, although examples of all the above purposes do exist. This non-decision-making emphasis is consistent with respect for a patient's rights, the physician's role, and the ultimate board accountability for patient care. The greater importance of educational programming over policy recommending suggests that the newness of this type of committee within the institutional structure, as well as the complexity of the issues it addresses, necessitates a heavy emphasis on educational activities aimed at solid grounding in the mission of the health care. For Catholic facilities, the ministry should be perceived as a faithful response to the Church's total mission; for nonsectarian institutions, a lived commitment to its corporate values.

Educational Activities

Consistent with the results of the CHA survey reported earlier in this work, each of the experienced panelists stressed education as the primary purpose of their committees. The entire workshop group, through written responses, also validated education as the principal purpose of institutional committees. The continued development of new medical technology, with its attendant ethical challenges, suggests the continued dominance of this purpose well into the 1990s. It was also generally agreed that educational activities must first be undertaken within the committee itself and then extended to staff, personnel, patients, family, and even the public, particularly legislators. The policy formation role emerges from the educational activity because new or deeper learnings frequently have as their final outcome the development or revision of policy. As committees mature, they also become more diversified and able to assume more activities.

Great diversity marks the current status of educational programming and services generated by hospital ethics committees. The activities reported by the panelists and participants include the following general categories and sample projects.

Ethical reflection. Within the framework of Christology and ecclesiology, individuals reflect on the meaning of the Church's mission, the health care ministry, and the person. This provides the context in which specific ethical issues are discussed from the theological, philosophical, and medical practice perspectives. In some cases the process is codified and serves as the basic method in which ethical issues are studied.

Study of the Ethical and Religious Directives for Catholic Health Facilities. The preamble of the *Directives,* as well as the specific directives on medical and religious practice, is presented to and discussed by board, management, physicians, nurses, and other staff. Stress is on the values and ethical principles on which the specific directives are based.

Forums. Forums are sponsored and conducted by experts to raise the consciousness level of employees and community members about the importance of specific clinical issues. Topics such as informed consent, confidentiality of information, family responsibilities, and new technologies such as low tubal ovum transfers and liver transplants are presented so that their ethical implications can be studied from different perspectives.

Orientation of new employees. New employees and new medical staff members are introduced to the facility's ethical posture as well as to the committee's existence and purpose. This is sometimes included in a presentation by a sponsoring group representative and includes a very general orientation to Catholic identity, congregational history and charism, and to the *Directives.*

Inservice education. The rationale for and elements of various policies (e.g., no code orders) are presented to employees to ensure understanding and proper implementation. Knowledge of the reasons for policies will assist in communication between physicians and other institutional personnel.

Patient and family counseling. Patients and families may be counseled about treatment options and their own responsibilities in decisions about care. This activity is only undertaken after the committee has matured in its functioning. The pastoral care and social services personnel play an important role in the referral process, but the attending physician must also be involved.

Staff counseling. Committees may also counsel institutional personnel and encourage physicians and nurses to view the committee and its members as a resource or sounding board for difficult situations or decisions. Quite obviously, again, this service is only possible when the committee has gained credibility within the institution.

Education for advocacy. One-on-one or group presentations may be offered to assist lawmakers, judges, lobbyists, and other public figures to understand issues so that their decisions are well informed. Such sessions should anticipate actual cases and be presented from the interdisciplinary perspective whenever possible.

Institutional and diocesan discernment. Institutional and diocesan representatives may discern issues through prayer, study of Scripture and Church teaching, review of the faithful's experience, and consultation with ethical, theological, and medical experts. Such sessions can be initiated by the sponsoring congregation, the administration, or the bishop.

Policy Activities

In addition to educational services, institutional ethics committees give high priority to reviewing and developing institutional policy. Many committees, in fact, initiate their committee activity by reviewing existing policies and recommending appropriate changes. Policies calling for immediate review generally include do-not-resuscitate (DNR) guidelines, termination of treatment protocols, recommendations for the care of severely handicapped infants, informed consent checklists, and guidelines for hyperalimentation and nasal gavage.

In implementing the policy review process, the committee generally studies the medical and ethical issues as well as the effectiveness of expression of the policy. After the preliminary study, the committee seeks broad consultation with the appropriate personnel. Many committees encourage ongoing contact with the same group of inhouse consultants throughout the policy review process. This ensures that decisions will be as valid as possible and that there will be great commitment to their implementation, particularly if existing policies are revised drastically. Such broad-based consultation can compensate for the limited size of a committee in comparison to the diversity of skills and size of staff as a whole. In the development of a new policy the same process of committee study and wide consultation is adopted to assure an adequate information base and personnel support.

Accountability and membership. The locus of accountability and the purpose of the committee both dictate its membership. Some committees are accountable to the board or to an overseeing board committee such as a patient care committee; some are accountable to the medical staff organization; others are accountable to administration or the chief executive officer (CEO). Although making the committee accountable to the board stresses its importance, making it accountable to the CEO makes its operation more efficient because of the opportunity for more immediate feedback. Making it accountable to the medical staff could play down the interdisciplinary approach to care even while it stresses physicians' responsibility. In making decisions about accountability and reporting mechanisms, one must be sensitive to both board and physician responsibility in regard to patient care.

These responsibilities, as well as the advantages and disadvantages of various types of committees, are presented in chart form at the end of this chapter.

Committee composition. A committee should generally have no fewer than 7 members and no more than 15. Consultants can be called in if an expertise not available within the committee is required by a specific situation. An interdisciplinary committee is generally considered more effective than a totally homogeneous group. There is also a distinct advantage in providing external community representation to an in-house committee. It is generally conceded that physicians, nurses, and patient counselors (clergy, pastoral care, social services) should be equally represented, although this may not be as appropriate when the committee is directly accountable to the medical staff organization. Physicians and nurses who are familiar with intensive care settings and physicians with a family practice orientation provide necessary expertise and experience. A psychiatrist is extremely helpful in hospice and long-term care settings. Although an attorney can provide helpful insights into the legal implications of a case or a policy, the hospital attorney is not the best choice, because he or she tends to have a defensive, litigation-conscious approach that can be counterproductive.

Elected officials, business leaders, former patients or family members, and local clergy are community members who should be given priority. It is also essential to have a Catholic moral theologian or ethicist *consistently* available, either as a committee member or as a consultant. To enhance communication with the diocese, it is also helpful to have a representative of the bishop as a committee member or as a consistent observer plus a member of the sponsoring group in institutions conducted by religious congregations. Because of the diversity of cultures represented in many urban hospitals and long-term care facilities, it is also desirable in those instances to have someone who has an intercultural orientation, such as an anthropologist or sociologist. Although this is desirable in all cases, it is essential if the committee takes on direct patient or family advising as one of its purposes.

Persons chosen for such committees must, first of all, be fully competent in their own fields. It is just as important to have high-level ethical and theological expertise available as it is to have high-level nursing and medical expertise. The range of medical expertise will necessarily increase and intensify if the committee involves itself in prognostic activities, although this committee function is not common. Committee members must also have a deep interest in the area of ethics and must be willing to commit the time required, not only for meetings but also for private study. They must also respect the need for confidentiality and practice it scrupulously. Because of the unique and complex nature of ethical issues, members must also be able to tolerate ambiguity and conflict. In addition, because such committees are also more process than task oriented, members must be able to sustain long discussions and perceived slowness in producing measurable results. The emphasis on committees' priority teaching role also suggests that members possess the ability to communicate information and facilitate learning. Even though formal affiliation with the Catholic Church is not necessary for all members and, in fact, is not always desirable because of the ecumenical nature of the service population, it is essential that all committee members share a faith vision and support the facility's commitment to Catholic ideals and moral teaching.

Operational guidelines. In addition to the overall guidelines of committee size of 7 to 15, panel participants at the workshop suggested other basic operational guidelines. Because of the complexity of issues referred to an ethics committee and the attendant need for study, it is deemed essential that appointment be for at least 2 and preferably 3 years, with staggered terms to provide for continuity. Carefully documented minutes are required, and, depending on the committee's purpose, notations of recommendations, referrals, and decisions should be made in the patient's individual record and in the permanent administration records. This is important for continuity of care as well as for liability documentation, even though no committee has thus far been held liable. In fact, insurance companies may provide, at no extra charge, committee coverage through a rider on the institution's liability policy because effective committees can, in fact, reduce risk and exposure.

Further suggestions on committee activities were offered by participants as operational guidelines. These can be categorized as attitudinal and process, although an overlap exists:

Attitudinal Suggestions

- Stress the fact that the committee work is process oriented and requires time and patient attention.

- Raise consciousness that interdisciplinary membership ("committee of experts") requires ongoing study in a variety of areas.

- Create an atmosphere for the committee and the entire institution that encourages ethical reflection.

- Recognize that some areas of the facility, such as neonatal intensive care, renal dialysis, and trauma centers, have greater problems and higher potential for both witness and counterwitness and may demand greater attention.

- Communicate purpose of committee clearly so that committee is not perceived as a "watchdog" or "institutional conscience."

- Emphasize the value of open, trusting relationship of physician, patient, and family as "preventive ethics."

Process Suggestions

- Anticipate issues so that committee is not responding to crises and time pressures, which reduce both effectiveness and efficiency.

- Schedule meetings monthly or bimonthly for 2-hour segments to allow for full discussion, and provide for effective preparation for meetings with agenda and supportive materials circulated well in advance.

- Discourage responding to beepers and plan meetings outside the facility or beyond the range of the intercom.

- Avoid both paternalism and elitism in manner of operating and transfer of traditional physician omniscience and omnipotence to the committee.

- Frequently identify the need for peer relationship so that intimidation by physicians, theologians, or ethicists is reduced.

- If the committee is to review cases, distinguish mandatory from optional ones and publish widely the criteria and method of referral.

- At outset, identify the interface of this committee with other in-house committees, such as quality assurance and Evaluative Criteria, and clearly articulate areas of responsibility and establish the manner of issue referral between committees.

- Distinguish between official Church teaching and speculative theology on specific issues so that the committee has a realistic understanding of guidelines.

- Determine if noninstitutional issues (e.g., medication for hospice and home care patients) should also be considered by the committee.

A wide range of models of institutional committees appears in the Appendixes, which further describe the manner in which committees function within the health care ministry.

Diocesan Committees

Purpose and function. The great diversity of the Catholic dioceses in the United States, the number of health care facilities, the availability of Catholic theologians and ethicists, and the extent of parish and diocesan involvement in the health ministry accounts for the great variety of diocesan committee models that have been implemented. There is one consistency, however. The committees that do exist attend to medical-moral issues only because other diocesan committees respond to the broader range of ethical subjects. Many diocesan committees have evolved to replace the individual priest consultant the bishop formerly depended on. The current tendency of the media to seek out episcopal opinions on medical-moral issues, however, is causing this role to appear again, with the bishop assembling and relying on a team of consultants rather than on one individual. Parallel to the purposes of institutional committees, the primary purpose of diocesan committees are advice on policy issues to the bishops or to the health care institutions within the diocese and educational programming for educational activities. In some cases the committees do appear to have decision-making powers and case review activities, but more frequently special cases that need diocesan consideration are referred directly to the bishop.

The underlying goal of the diocesan committees, no matter the purpose, appears to be achieving unity and consistency in implementing the *Ethical and Religious Directives* and effective communication among the various constituencies concerned with health. The value of unity for stronger public policy advocacy is also recognized. In addition, the diocesan committee may focus on the medical-moral education of the clergy as the basis for broader education in Church teaching. To assist the laity in formation of conscience, the committee may develop programs that relate the medical and theological aspects of issues commonly encountered in health care. These can be then implemented at the diocesan, deanery, or parish levels.

As an alternative to an ongoing committee, some bishops have ad hoc groups they convene to deal with specific issues and questions; thus the membership will vary from group to group. At times, the individuals involved in a specific case appear before this ad hoc group. This alternative can be used when the bishop wishes to explore the problem of scandal caused by proposed collaborative arrangements of a Catholic facility with an individual or instituion not acting in a manner consistent with Catholic-Christian norms. It can also be used when the bishop needs assistance in responding to proposed legislation such as living will bills, fetal research, and Medicaid eligibility standards.

Accountability and membership. Because of the bishop's role as the interpreter of Church teaching, a diocesan committee is ultimately accountable to him. The committee, then, is a consultative body with no decision-making powers, while an intermediary such as the diocesan ethicist or the health care coordinator serves as the linkage between the bishop and the committee.

In terms of membership, two general models prevail. In each model the number of members is relatively larger than on the institutional committees. This reflects the need to respond to the diverse diocesan constituencies, although some very small committees or groups do exist in large dioceses. The first model is institution specific and includes interdisciplinary representation for each of the Catholic facilities in the diocese as well as diocesan staff and general public representatives. The second model is formed without reference to the individual institutions, although some members will, of course, be affiliated with the facilities In some cases the bishop serves on the committee; in others, he is not involved directly but receives the recommendations and decisions from the committee through the intermediary mentioned above. It is significant that diocesan committees have more theologians, philosophers, and physicians as members than do institutional committees, although nurses, family representatives, and attorneys are also represented. In several cases where legislative vigilance is a defined purpose, the membership composition will also reflect this special interest.

Although diocesan committees are generally large, the size of the actual committee varies from just 5 members in one very large diocese to over 30 members in another diocese where every health care institution has representation. In some cases where the committee is small, efforts are made to contact the administrators of the health care facilities before developing the agenda for the monthly meeting. Some small committees also function through ad hoc subcommittee structure. For specific issues they either expand their membership as required by the concern or form a new subcommittee to address the issue.

Operational guidelines. The great diversity that marks the diocesan committees precludes specific operational guidelines beyond some very basic observations. Diocesan committees generally meet on an ad hoc, monthly, or quarterly basis. Although minutes are maintained, those dealing with specific cases remain confidential, with summaries distributed to members. Often diocesan media publicize the committees' educational activities and publish a summary report of committee activities in the diocesan paper. Tenure on the diocesan committee ranges from two to three years, with appointment directly by the bishop being the most common method of appointment.

One of the more important issues raised by the diocesan committee is the communication network required to keep all those involved in diocesan health care apprised of recommendations and decisions. This is particularly difficult in a diocese where the health care facilities are numerous and varied and are sponsored by various congregations who may have their own committees in place, both at the institutional and system level. There is consensus that the potential for diocesan collaboration has not been adequately realized, although more are becoming aware of the necessity for coordinating activities, particularly educational ones. The ethics committee becomes the obvious focus for planning and executing such diocesan-wide activities. The growing trend of appointing a diocesan or regional consultant in medical ethics may facilitate this type of communication and collaboration.

The various models of diocesan ethics committees in the back of this book reflect the great diversity that currently marks them.

Multi-institutional System Committees

At present, at the multi-institutional system level, the corporate ethicist is a far more common phenomenon than the ethics committee. There is also a tendency at the corporate level to adopt a more global ethical approach and encompass issues of management, labor relations, and allocation of resources as well as clinical practice, under committee activity or the corporate resource person. Whether the modality is the individual ethicist or the ethics committee, however, the major emphasis at the corporate level is fourfold: motivation, education, networking, and monitoring. The overall purpose of the ethicist and the committee is simply to encourage ethical reflection as a priority at the local level and to provide centrally the resources and specialized expertise not available at the individual institutions. The centralization also allows for controlled experimentation with a variety of models as well as for exchange of information, experiences, and personnel.

The following example of the motivational role of the corporate ethicist is typical. The corporate ethicist, or human values coordinator, as some are called, visits the member institutions and, during an ethical reflection week, meets with small interdisciplinary groups of 10 to 12 persons during all three shifts. During these sessions he or she facilitates discussions on values, on the congregational charism, and on ethical decision making. This activity helps in establishing a climate for the formation of an institutional committee and provides a core experience for all institutions within a system that serves as a common base for subsequent activities.

The ethicist at the corporate level also plans and implements educational activities such as forum and in-service programs. Although these sometimes involve the corporate board and the local board, more frequently they are limited to the local personnel. The corporate ethicist develops such programs and takes them on the road to sponsored facilities. This precludes the necessity for local staffing and unifies the corporate ministry within the system.

Although not currently in place, two model system committees that provide medical-moral direction to member institutions are described in the Appendix. The first model operates out of the corporate headquarters, and membership does not specifically reflect the institutions within the system. Because the institutions in a multihospital system are generally in several dioceses, this committee, with its centralized authority, may experience some difficulty in relating its activity to that of the various dioceses Despite this, the method does assist the sponsoring congregation in its accountability efforts In such a model the corporate committee develops guidelines and policies, which are then referred to the institution for implementation Unless the institutions within the system are similar, this may require a very wide range of expertise at the corporate level. In this model, the committee is required to meet regularly and must establish effective communication from the corporate headquarters to each facility.

In the second model, the primary purpose is communication and networking. This committee is composed of representatives of each of the institutions within the system. In this model the local, not the corporate, board would be the policy making group, but the committee would become a clearing house for experiences and activities. In this model, meetings are generally held just once or twice a year.

Because of the newness of multihospital systems and the increasing emphasis on congregational and diocesan responsibility, this type of committee will undoubtedly become more popular, as will the corporate ethicist.

Model Institutional Committee

On the following pages appear a brief summation of the advantages and disadvantages of various types of committees as well as a model of a fictional ethics committee. This model has been developed from the presentation and participants' discussions at the ethics workshop. The editors have preferred to present it in a descriptive form rather than formal organizational bylaw format to allow for greater ease of interpretation and adaptation. It conforms to the principles identified at the beginning of this chapter, and it concentrates its efforts on educational programming and policy development. These two functions appear most consistent with the current status of committees and the other relationships established within the health care facility. Although focused on the institutional committee and appropriate for either an acute or long-term care facility, the concepts and structure of the proposed model can easily be adapted to the diocese or even the system.

In addition, the models and the job descriptions described in the back of this book will also suggest other functions and operational guidelines that can be adapted for various uses.

Types of Ethics Committees

Committee Type*	Advantages	Disadvantages
Institutional		
Board		
Committee is composed of board members only.	Board is ultimately accountable for patient care and policy decisions.	Board members generally do not have range of expertise to deal with issues.
Administration		
Committee is composed of persons who serve in administrative roles within facility, including administration of medical staff.	Members are familiar with institutional philosophy and goals and are accountable to board for liability issues.	Individuals in group are involved with a large number of committees and in most cases are removed from patient issues.
Medical Staff		
Committee is composed exclusively of medical staff members, although CEO may be ex-officio.	Issues are clinical, and physicians have expertise and are accountable to and for the patients.	Medical aspect is basic but only one phase of ethical decision making.
Interdisciplinary (intrainstitutional)		
Persons represent various	Persons affiliated with	Nearness to situation can

Committee Type*	Advantages	Disadvantages
disciplines but all come from within the institution itself (board, physicians, employees).	institutions have greater familiarity with issues and are directly concerned with outcome.	influence objectivity and can preclude healthy challenges from outside.
Interdisciplinary (intraextrainstitutional)		
Committee is composed of persons representing various disciplines who are both within the institution but also external to it, such as diocesan representatives, patients, local clergy, family members, community members.	External representation provides important observations for persons not directly responsible to the institution but directly involved with its image and services.	Persons external to health care often need some orientation and instruction in health issues.
Diocesan		
General		
Committee is composed of various persons within the diocese. It can include representatives of the health care institutions but membership is not determined by health care involvement.	Unifies ministry at the diocesan level and allows for broad representation from general community and ecclesial circles.	Lack of direct involvement with individual institutions and lack of opportunity for relationship with them can affect quality of discussion as well as communication.

*Membership described above is limited to voting members and does not preclude advisory groups to the committee.

Types of Ethics Committees

Committee Type*	Advantages	Disadvantages
Institution Oriented Committee is composed of various persons within the diocese, but structure and membership has been developed to ensure adequate representation of all health care within the diocese.	Provides effective networking between local Church and institutions as well as among health care institutions.	In large diocese with several and varied facilities, committee could be unmanageable and diffuse.
System *Corporate* Committee is composed of persons at the corporate level of the system.	Easier to convene individuals and to unify activities and take action quickly.	Development of policy away from site of implementation can diminish institutional commitment.
Corporate and Interinstitutional Committee is composed of persons at the corporate level but also of representatives of each of the institutions within the system.	Allows for more communication and discussion of issues between persons who are involved with the issues firsthand and those who hold final accountability.	Distance generally precludes the frequency of meetings required for cycle of study-discussion-development-orientation-implementation.

*Membership described above is limited to voting members and does not preclude advisory groups to the committee.

Proposed Model
Christian Medical Ethics Committee
Good News Health Center
Utopia, ZA

Purpose

The Christian medical ethics committee at Good News Health Center is established to provide a forum for the discussion of ethical issues and the development of policies and educational programming for the facility (staff, personnel, patients, and families) and the community. It is ultimately accountable to the board of trustees and will maintain this accountability through the CEO to the chairman of the board. The committee will carry on its deliberations in the light of Good News Health Center's commitment to uphold the medical-moral ideals and principles of the Catholic Church and the stewardship obligations of the sponsoring group and the diocesan bishop. The committee provides an interdisciplinary forum for the study of the reflection on Church teaching as it applies to health issues. It will emphasize medical issues and not deliberate on social justice questions.

Functions

The committee's functions are listed below:

1. To contribute to an institutional climate in which ethical reflection can occur

2. To review clinical policies and make recommendations about their moral appropriateness

3. To review and make recommendations on policies and procedures involving general patient and family rights in regard to admission and treatment

4. To collaborate with other institutional divisions in providing an ethical component to medical rounds and other educational activities

5. To recommend educational programs in the area of Christian medical ethics for board, personnel (orientation and in-service), patients, and community

6. To serve as a resource to administrator, physicians and nurses, and other personnel who wish to consult about issues of patient care within the institution (but committee does not make decisions on specific cases)

7. To identify possible future problems so that appropriate study will allow the institution to respond proactively

8. To collaborate within the facility so that timely articles on ethical issues appear regularly in institutional publications

9. To provide periodic reports to the board on the ethical situation within the institution.

10. To conduct retrospective reviews of management of specific clinical cases when requested by institutional managers.

Membership

The CEO will recommend persons to this committee, and the board of trustees will appoint the membership, which shall not be fewer than 9 and not more than 15. Before recommending members, the CEO (who may serve on the committee) should ascertain individuals' interest in the subject as well as their willingness to contribute the necessary time for meetings and study. Efforts should be made to gain diversity of competence and experience. At least three fourths of the members must be part of the institutional community, with the other fourth representing the diocese and the general community. The following categories of persons should be represented:

Administration
Medical staff
Nursing personnel
Pastoral care personnel
Lawyer (not institutional attorney)

Clergy
Social services personnel
Catholic moral theologian
Representative of sponsoring
group and of diocese

Terms

Each member will serve for three years and may be reappointed for three additional years. To provide continuity, one third of the committee will be rotated annually.

Officers

The CEO will appoint the chairperson of the committee, and the members will elect their own secretary. Both the chairperson and the secretary will serve for one year; but after a year out of office they may again hold the same office.

Operational Guidelines

Operational guidelines are as follows:

1. For orientation purposes, all committee members are required to read materials cited on the general committee resource list so that all come to meetings with a common educational base.

2. Meetings are held at least monthly, generally for two hours and as needed to address special issues.

3. Although it is recommended that consensus rather than actual voting be the usual mode of coming to decision, no decision made by the committee may be considered a valid recommendation unless three-fourths of the committee members are present for a vote and 75 percent of the members present approve it.

4. Minutes of the meeting are forwarded to the Good News Health Center administration within 2 weeks of each meeting. If a particular case is referred to the committee for review prospectively and retrospectively, a notation of that review is placed in the appropriate record and file. The CEO forwards copies of minutes to the diocesan bishop or the representative he has designated and to the sponsoring group.

5. All deliberations of the committees are considered confidential.

6. To provide for specialized study, the committee may expand its membership by appointing subcommittees or by having resource persons participate in meetings. Such subcommittees and resource persons should not have an actual vote in decision making, although their opinions on issues can and should be solicited.

7. Chairperson of committee will meet quarterly with CEO and chairperson of institutional quality assurance education, and Christian effectiveness committees to share information and coordinate activities as required.

Discussion

Question: Is it not necessary to avoid "clericalism" on committees by having some grass roots people as well as persons from other denominations? Don't we need to profit from the personal prayer and reflection of many while not denying theologians' expertise?

Panelist: Theologians need the scientific basis and background that only medical personnel can give. We would get no place without seeing that many physicians of all faiths are willing to provide it. In fact, as committees work with physicians and family members and others, it becomes apparent that few differences exist because of the shared concern for the person and human values. We all must depend on prayer when we are dealing with ethical issues, *especially* the theologians.

Panelist: The grass roots input is the real value of having current or former patients or patients' family members on committees.

Question: Is some of the recent emphasis on forming committees the result of religious congregations' fearing they are losing control as their numbers decrease?

Panelist: It appears rather to be a reflection of the greater seriousness of the ethical issues and the effect of rapidly advancing technology, the aging population, and economic cutbacks, all of which will force ethical decisions. It also is a bit of preventive medicine, because in 1973, when the Supreme Court made its decision on *Roe V. Wade*, we found we had not prepared as well as we might have. There is also a general tendency in health care and in the Church now to be more proactive than reactive. In the legal sense, ethics committees can be part of an institution's risk management program—preventive law as well as preventive medicine.

Question: Can members of ethics committees be sued?

Panelist: Ethics committees are exposed to liability under existing law in all 50 states plus Guam and the Phillipines. Since this presentation, legislation has been passed in Louisiana and introduced in other states which protects the records and proceedings of hospital ethics committees and protects both committee members and those persons presenting information to the committee. However, insurance agents generally react favorably when shown that the committee is a way to reduce exposure to civil and criminal liability. This, of course, carries the expectation of a reduction in the existing premium, analogous to a nonsmoker getting a reduction in life insurance. In cases that I am familiar with, a rider was extended to cover the ethics committee and no additional premium was levied. In the context of a modern, American lawsuit, each individual on an ethics committee, as well as the institution within which it functions, is a conceivable target or defendant in lawsuits. An agreement by the hospital to indemnify and hold harmless the ethics committee members, coupled with insurance, should remove any possibility of personal liability even if committee members were named as defendents.

Question: The ethical methodology of proportionalism has been presented here in an unfavorable light. Is this just and accurate?

Panelist: There is a legitimate diversity of opinion in moral theology today. Vatican II called for a renewal of moral theology, and we are in an exploratory era. The two conferences of bishops in North America reflect this diversity, since the American bishops in their *Directives* refer to the administrator's obligation to ensure that the directives are followed, while the Canadian bishops have issued Guidelines to assist physicians and patients in their conscientious decision making.

Panelist: I am not proportionalist, but I think the proportionalists have contributed to progress in moral theology, especially in calling our attention more and more to the dignity of the person and the need to pay attention to that dignity in making moral judgments. Where the proportionalists can help in the development of moral theology in the Church is on the speculative level, in that discernment process that Abp. Pilarczyk spoke of. I quarrel mainly with the proportionalists in that they tend to speak as if their theory can be followed in practice when it differs from the Church's magisterial teaching. On this they do a disservice to the progress of moral theology and to the Church.

Question: What would the relationship be between the *Evaluative Criteria* project (of which I am the chairperson) and a human values committee or an ethics committee? Unless this is clarified, there could be frustration, confusion, and duplication of efforts.

Panelist: As you know, principle 5 of the *Evaluative Criteria for Health Care Facilities* relates to medical-moral guidance. In its five guidelines, it calls for carefully articulated ethical policies and procedures, a structured decision-making process, provision of ethical guidance, qualified staff advisors in the area of ethics, and a broad range of educational programming. The institutional ethics committee could assume responsibility for that particular chapter within the overall *Evaluative Criteria* project.

Panelist: In our institution, we have an ethical consultant who is a moral theologian and an interdisciplinary subcommittee of the *Evaluative Criteria* project that meets and works on principle 5. The basic values that are dealt with in this principle appear throughout the document, so that discussion will have the same focus in various *Criteria* committees, but the application will be specific to the principle.

Panelist: In our institutions, when we met initially to decide if we needed an ethics committee, we used the Evaluative Criteria principle 5 to determine what our committee should look for and if we should even have a committee. Now we periodically go back and evaluate ourselves on that criterion. Our Evaluative Criteria committee is dealing with the eight criteria one by one with separate committees, so we have adopted responsibility for that one criteria.

Question: As a sociologist, I would like to recommend another type of member for the committee. I urge strongly that those of us at hospitals with a very heterogeneous population recognize that diversity. It is not uncommon in a Brooklyn emergency room to hear six languages being spoken simultaneously. Haitian Catholicism, for example, is culturally different from Hispanic and Anglo Catholicism. When you talk about people who compose these committees, I think it is critical that there be someone who is sensitive to religious and cultural differences. When you put religion through the funnel of culture, it has different results.

Panelist: That is a very good observation. In addition, I would like to suggest having an elected official on the committee to gain the community, nonhealth, professional viewpoint.

Question: What is the difference between a medical-moral committee and a medical-ethics committee?

Panelist: Ethics is a reflection on what is appropriate and inappropriate in human action drawn from observations of human reason. Moral theology brings to that process the data of positive revelation. In a Catholic hospital, then, we often speak of a medical-moral committee as emphasizing Christian morality and Catholic teaching, rather than of a strict medical-ethics committee, because there is an added source of light on the problem, namely, divine revelation. (These terms are distinguished more fully in the glossary of terms which appears in the final section of this book.)

Question: In a situation where there currently is no committee at the institutional or the diocesan level, would it not be advisable to have a diocesan think tank model that would then send policies and so on to the institutions? It would be a bit like the diocesan committee being the main computer and every Catholic hospital having a terminal to deal with its own specific questions.

Panelist: Our situation is different because we have no Catholic hospitals in the diocese, so the diocesan model has far greater importance in educating the people and representing the Christian view to the nondenominational facilities. People do agree that there is benefit in having unity in the approach through the National Catholic Health Office, and we agreed that there should be one medical-moral code.

Panelist: We must be realistic about the amount of time that any bishop can give to this project, and we should try to implement the principle of subsidiarity. The particular area for mutuality is that reflection process that has been talked about.

Question: I still wonder whether the committee should focus on medical-moral problems, clinical questions, or go beyond these issues to labor-management relationships, justice in investments, outreach programs for the poor, and so on.

Panelist. I recommend that the committee be a medical-moral committee and deal with that aspect of Catholic identity. The *Evaluative Criteria* document lists all the issues you raise, and our institution has approached them through that document but kept the medical-moral committee strictly medical-moral.

Panelist: We have tried both models. In one hospital we are now integrating the medical-moral and in another the social justice emphasis, and we will watch those carefully. My own sense is that because of the short history of committees, we probably should start with medical-moral issues; however, conceptually I do not think that is the better way, because when we reflect on medical-moral issues we are talking about doing justice to people. The Church has clearly said that justice is a constitutive part of the Gospel and our mission. The more we can integrate the social justice dimension into the institution's everyday life in the way we relate to patients and employees, the more whole we will become as an institution. We also must keep the business dimension integrated. To use an analogy, the ethical dimension is the central strand in the cable of health ministry, whether it be patient care, employee relations, or use of resources.

Question: As a legislator, I would like to affirm the stress that has been laid on the importance of educating and involving persons from the political arenas in ethical discussion.

Question: As one who has lived through strikes and has tried to live out the justice issues in labor relations and other challenges, I would like to suggest that in our work with committees we seek out the contemplative communities as a source of prayerful support.

Question: Where does the Catholic Church stand in terms of its Catholic hospitals? Is there a commitment from the hierarchy to maintain Catholic facilities?

Panelist: Although the lack of vocations has caused some congregations to close their hospitals, I am sure the bishops want to back us up and do what they can to keep a hospital Catholic.

Panelist: Part of the answer to the question lies in the fact that in 1981, the American bishops affirmed their support for Catholic facilities in their pastoral "On Health and Health Care." They also affirmed this in a survey conducted among bishops by The Catholic Health Association in 1982. The Canadian bishops are currently preparing a health pastoral, and that draft suggests their very strong support of involvement in institutional care.

Part Four
References and Resources

Models of Institutional Ethics Committees

Sample

Institutional Model 1

Institutional Medical-Moral Review Committee

The medical-moral committee shall consist of no fewer than six persons appointed by the chairman of the board of directors. Two of the persons shall be members of the medical-dental staff, two shall be members of the board of directors, one shall be a person knowledgeable in moral theology, and one shall be the CEO of the hospital. This committee, which shall meet monthly, shall have the responsibility to review special medical procedures and practices to ensure that the hospital is faithful to the implementation of the moral directives as promulgated by the National Conference of Catholic Bishops (NCCB).

Sample

Institutional Model 2

Institutional Medical-Moral Committee

Key Objective

To provide a mechanism for understanding and interpreting Church teaching on medical-moral issues through interdisciplinary dialogue, resulting in appropriate recommendations when medical-moral issues are involved.

Critical Objectives

To provide an open interdisciplinary forum for discussion of pertinent medical-moral issues as they relate to the medical center.

Standards

1. Members of the committee named by the administrator represent administration, medical staff, nursing staff, pastoral care personnel, and the community.

2. Committee members are informed about and educated in medical-moral matters, the health care objectives of the sponsoring congregation, and Church teaching.

3. The committee reviews and makes recommendations as needed on cases where medical-moral issues are involved.

4. The committee actively supports appropriate medical-moral education throughout the medical center.

5. The committee is convened by the administrator as needed.

Sample

Institutional Model 3

Board Committee on Ethical Responsibility

Definition

The committee on ethical responsibility is a standing committee of the board of trustees. Appointments to standing committees are made annually for a term of one year. The president of the board of trustees makes these appointments as soon as possible after the board of trustees' annual meeting.

Purpose

The purpose of the committee on ethical responsibility is to assist the board in developing, confirming, and communicating policies related to ethical responsibility.

Authority

With the exception of reserved powers as specified, the corporate member has delegated total authority and responsibility to the board of trustees for the operation of the Catholic facility in accordance with the congregation's policies for corporate organization and in compliance with the *Ethical and Religious Directives for Catholic Health Facilities.*

Membership

Composition

At least three members of the committee must be members of the board of trustees. Other members are appointed. The executive director is an ex-officio member of all committees. Membership should include a physician, a registered nurse, a member of the sponsoring congregation, one or both executive administrators, and a moral theologian or ethicist.

Qualifications

- Interest in serving the board in the area of ethical responsibility
- Ability to set aside time to broaden and deepen personal knowledge in the area of ethical responsibility through private study and attendance at workshops, institutes, and continuing education courses

Responsibilities

- To review and reinforce the hospital's basic commitment to ethical values, with particular emphasis on conforming to the congregation's policies for corporate organization, the philosophy for health care services conducted under the auspices of the Sisters, and the *Ethical and Religious Directives for Catholic Health Facilities*

- To educate its members and all board members about ethical responsibility

- To recommend to the board the establishment, clarification, confirmation, and communication of ethical policy and to take responsibility for formulating ethical policies according to prescribed norms, as listed in no. 1 above

- To advise hospital management on internal medical-moral decisions and to receive and evaluate reports of medical-moral decisions reached

- To serve as resource persons and to monitor the hospital's program of ethical education, which is intended to develop understanding and acceptance at all levels

- To advise the board and the CEO on resource allocation specifically related to ethical responsibility

- To give ongoing assurance to the board on the acceptable quality of hospital response to questions of ethics, the overall institutional moral tone, and total patient well-being

Meetings

The committee shall meet 10 times each year or more frequently as called by the chairman.

Recommendation

A moral theologian should be contracted with to assist the committee.

| Sample |

Institutional Model 4

Institutional Medical-Moral Committee

Nature and Purpose

Rather than being a watchdog or a policy-recommending group, the committee is a study and research group. It seeks a fuller understanding of the reasons underlying certain ethical positions of the Catholic Church, recognizes the limitations and ambiguity of issues, and relates the data of medical practice to Christian values. It conducts ongoing study of relevant ethical problems, weighs alternative viewpoints, and renders opinions if requested. In this way, the committee is representative of Catholic educational and research tradition and makes a modest contribution, at least in-house, to the understanding of current medical-moral problems. In due course, this understanding can be communicated in appropriate ways to the hospital's health care personnel.

The purposes of the committee are thus as follows:

- To facilitate study and communication on ethical problems among the various competencies concerned with patient care

- To develop a sensitivity to fundamental human values as they relate to the Christian tradition and total patient care

- To educate committee members and, in turn, other members of the health care community to trends in medical-moral problems

- To offer counsel and opinions on questions proposed for study by the administration or appropriate hospital departments.

Membership

The committee should be composed of 8 to 10 persons directly involved in patient care and who at the same time have an active interest in ethical issues. The following departments should be represented: medical and scientific staff, nursing, patient and family counseling, diagnostic and treatment center, administration, pastoral care. Around the core group, adjunct members who bring a particular expertise to the question under study can be added at a given time. These might include a moral theologian, a medical specialist, legal counsel, and the like. Members serve for 2 years, renewable for a second term if the president of the hospital so chooses.

Sample

Institutional Model 5

Ethical Issues Forum

Purpose

The ethical issues forum is an advisory committee that serves as a resource to administration and staff in clarifying ethical issues arising out of the modern practice of medicine within the framework of the institution's philosophy.

Functions

- To review and discuss "ethical issues" literature for self-education and to assist in developing educational programs for medical, nursing, and allied health personnel in the field of bioethics

- To provide a forum for interdisciplinary dialogue and exchange on ethical principles

- To monitor legislation and relevant legal proceedings in an effort to determine the ethical consequences of legal developments in the field of bioethics

- To serve as a resource for the medical, nursing, and allied health staff and patients and families in dealing with ethical questions related to treatment

- To serve as an advisory body to administration and the professional staff on the formulation of policy and guidelines related to ethical issues in health care.

Membership

Members will be selected by the president and CEO or CEO designate for a two-year appointment. Half the members will be replaced in two years.

Medical Staff Representatives

- Neurology or neurosurgery

- Oncology

- Neonatology

- Internal medicine or cardiology

- General surgery or family medicine

Nursing Staff Representatives

- Critical care or intermediate critical care

- Nursery

- Oncology or hospice

- Medical

- Emergency room

- Support Services Representatives

- Pastoral Care

- Social Services

- Respiratory Therapy

Administration Representatives
Consumer Representatives

Meetings

Meetings will be held monthly. A representative of the committee is to be available for consultation to the staff on a 24-hour basis.

Minutes

Minutes with recommendations will be forwarded to the president
and CEO. Confidentiality of physicians, staff, patients, and family
who choose to use the committee as a resource will be maintained.
The minutes will include a summary of any cases presented
without identifying names of staff, patients, or families.

Reporting Relationship

The ethical issues forum is an administrative committee
reporting to the president and CEO. Recommendations may be
referred to the executive committee of the medical staff or other
staff committees at the discretion of the president and CEO.

Sample

Institutional Model 6

Institutional Ethics Committee

Function

Because of the increasingly complex nature of medical
decision making and the ethical concerns that arise in health care
institutions today, the hospital ethics committee was formed to
provide guidance in addressing these concerns. The hospital has
an obligation and a need to establish, confirm, and communicate
ethical policies. The hospital also is responsible for ensuring that
all levels of the organization are properly educated to understand
and accept these ethical policies as essential to their hospital
relationships. As a Catholic hospital, the hospital's ethical
responsibilities are of utmost importance.

Purpose

- To provide a forum for interdisciplinary dialogue on ethical and
  moral questions arising in the hospital

- To advise hospital administration and professional staff in formulating medical-moral guidelines consistent with Catholic values

- To monitor legislative changes that may have medical-moral implications

- To educate the hospital and the community it serves in developing medical moral trends in effective health care

Authority

The board of trustees has authorized the hospital ethics committee to fulfill its stated purpose. The chairperson, on behalf of the committee, shall make formal recommendations to the board of trustees, the CEO, or both, who are responsible for authorizing the committee or various other departments within the hospital to act on these recommendations.

Membership and Committee Structure

Membership on the hospital ethics committee is granted by appointment of the board of trustees. Representatives from the medical staff shall be appointed by the president of the medical staff. Membership becomes effective upon acceptance. Membership on the committee shall be for two years and may be reviewed by appointment for two additional years.

Committee membership shall consist of the following:

- A minimum of two members of the board of trustees

- A minimum of three representatives of the medical-dental staff

- CEO or executive vice president

- Vice president of nursing and patient care

- Vice president of finance

- Department manager of pastoral services

- Department manager of social services

- Two community representatives

- Director of legal services

- An outside consultant for Theology/Ethics*

- Executive Secretary*

- Educational resources coordinator

*Ex-officio members

Operational Guidelines

Officers

The officers of the hospital ethics committee shall be chairperson and vice chairperson. These officers will be appointed by the board of trustees for a one-year term each.

The chairperson shall do as follows:

- Be a representative from the board of trustees

- Call and preside at all general meetings

- Be accountable to the board of trustees for the quality and efficiency of the service and performance of the hospital ethics committee

- Appoint any standing committees or subcommittees as necessary and designate the chairperson for these committees

The vice-chairperson shall do as follows:

- Assume the duties of the chairperson in the absence of that officer

- Perform duties assigned by the chairperson. Two members (the executive secretary and the educational resources coordinator) will act as staff to the committee

The executive secretary shall do as follows:

- Keep accurate minutes of the committee meetings and distribute the minutes to the members within two weeks after a Committee meeting

- Send a notice of meetings, including agenda, to the members approximately two weeks before the next meeting

The educational resources coordinator shall do as follows:

- Coordinate all aspects of the hospital ethics committee

- Be responsible for the agenda for all general meetings

- Provide any necessary research for the committee

- Be available to make any necessary contracts outside the hospital as well as serve on any necessary ad hoc committees

- Carry out the committee's educational directives in the hospital and in the community

Meetings

Meetings will be held quarterly or as determined by the chairperson. Members are to be available on an ad hoc basis as circumstances require.

Quorum

At least half the committee members must be present to constitute a quorum for a meeting.

Models of Diocesan Ethics Committees

| Sample |

Diocesan Model 1

Diocesan Medical-Moral Committee

The diocesan medical-moral committee will serve as a communication and advisory group linking the health care facilities of the diocese with the bishop.

Purposes

- To provide a forum for sharing concerns and information on medical-moral subjects

- To provide a forum for discussing application of the *Ethical and Religious Directives for Catholic Health Facilities* and magisterial teaching in medical-moral areas

- To seek to develop a unified stance on particular issues within the diocese

- To advise the bishop on issues where an episcopal statement is desired or needed

- To plan one major educational program in ethics each year for all persons involved in health care in the diocese

Committee Membership

In addition to the five members of the committee appointed by the bishop, each health care facility within the diocese may name two persons to the committee. To ensure appropriate representation, the bishop may also appoint three other persons to the committee after the initial appointments are made. Each person may serve on the committee for three years and then may not serve for two years. Terms are arranged so that a third of the institutions make appointments every third year.

Guidelines

- The committee meets at least nine times a year.

- The chairperson of the committee is elected annually from a list of three nominees submitted by a subcommittee and approved by the bishop. The bishop or his designate and the chairperson plan agenda for each meeting.

- Committee reports are included in diocesan reports, but the minutes are not circulated beyond the committee membership. (This is to allow for complete freedom in dealing with sensitive issues.)

- Any individual within the diocese may refer an ethical issue to the committee for advice, but all decision making will follow regular lines of authority and accountability at the appropriate levels.

- At the invitation of the chairperson, experts in various fields may participate in committee meetings at any time but without the right to vote.

- The committee may appoint subcommittees to deal with specific topics, but any recommendation to the bishop must be approved by two thirds of the entire committee.

Sample

Diocesan Model 2

Diocesan Medical-Moral Board

Responsibilities

- To be a resource in the areas of moral and ethical concerns

- To promote and coordinate workshops in the area of bioethical and moral concerns and to assist the health facilities to develop programs of orientation to the policies of a particular hospital and the principles of the Church on medical-moral issues

- To serve as a facilitator in matters of pastoral or bioethical concerns that call for expertise outside the health care facility itself

The medical-moral board functions under the direction of its chairman, who is responsible to the secretary of social ministry of the archdiocese.

Purposes

Education

The main task of the board is to assume responsibility for educating the total hospital community on the nature and purpose of a Catholic health care facility. This includes insights into the hospital as a healing community, the basic Christian values to which it gives witness, and methods of implementing these values. Through a program of orientation, lecture, discussion, workshop, conference, and other educative devices, the board's task is to further the ongoing process of moral development and medical-moral formation within the entire hospital community. The board always carries out this task in consultation with the hospital itself.

Printed with permission of the Archdiocese of San Francisco.

The emphasis on particular decisions is not as important as is developing a sense of fundamental values that guide the day-to-day operation of the Catholic hospital.

Inderdisciplinary Dialogue

A second purpose of the board is to provide a forum for interdisciplinary dialogue and exchange. The decisions that hospitals face are so complex that interdisciplinary thought is demanded, yet few forums exist whereby health care providers can gather and discuss areas relative to human and ethical values in health affairs. The medical-moral board provides this interdisciplinary forum for identifying and clarifying key ethical issues and for recommending policies if necessary.

Unity

A third purpose of the board is to provide a basis for unity within and among the Catholic health facilities in the understanding and application of Catholic moral principles. This is necessary in the midst of increasing ambiguity and complexity of medical-moral issues. In addition, the medical-moral board helps to ensure among the personnel of the Catholic health facilities a sense of unity in interpretation and implementation of hospital policy and of the *Ethical and Religious Directives for Catholic Health Facilities.*

Channel of Communication

The board serves as a channel of communication from the line of experience to the line of policy making. Hospital personnel, working through the hospital's own lines of administration, can bring ethical issues to the board's attention. The board thus provides a forum where the ethical dimensions of health care are surfaced and alternatives raised.

Legislative Vigilance

The board desires to be sensitive to the moral implications of state and federal legislation as it affects the health care apostolate; monitoring legal implications in this area is itself a tremendous task and responsibility.

Membership of Board

The chairman of the board is appointed by the archbishop. The length of time of this appointment is for the archbishop to decide. The board will number never fewer than five nor more than eight members not counting the chairman. Board members serve for a term of 2 years and may serve for two consecutive terms. At no time will all board members leave office concomitantly. Recommendation for board membership is made by current board members in consultation with the archdiocesan secretary of social ministry of the archdiocese. The archbishop ultimately approves and appoints board members. Rotation of board members will take place at the first meeting after October 1. Board members will serve as secretary for meetings on a rotating basis.

Guidelines

The medical-moral board functions in this manner:

Meetings

The board will meet regularly once every other month at a place and time designated by the board itself. The board will also meet on an ad hoc basis when some need arises. The chairman of the board will draw up the agenda for meetings in consultation with board members and the administrators of the Catholic health facilities. Administration and staff members of the health facilities should always feel free to contact any member of the board for consultation and for agenda items for board meetings.

Subcommittees

Should a special need arise, the board may appoint a subcommittee to study and research a specific topic or area of concern. Such a subcommittee is directly responsible to the board. Its membership and duration depend on the board's discretion.

Sample

Diocesan Model 3

Constitution
of the
Medical Ethics Commission
Diocese of Richmond

Article 1
Name and Purpose

The name of the commission shall be the medical ethics commission, diocese of Richmond. The purpose of the commission is as follows:

1. To identify the critical medical moral issues facing the diocese in the delivery of health care

2. To study those issues as they relate to the *Ethical and Religious Directives for Catholic Health Facilities* and with the advice of outside consultants

3. To study the *Ethical and Religious Directives for Catholic Health Facilities* and the issues to which they speak in order to gain a better understanding of them and their implementation

4. To make recommendations to the bishop on critical medical-moral issues and the *Ethical and Religious Directives for Catholic Health Facilities*

Article II
Membership

The membership of the commission shall be composed of no more than twenty (20) members and no more than ten (10) associate members. Members shall be appointed annually by the bishop for a term of one year and may serve successive terms.

Members shall be drawn from the administrative staffs, pastoral care staffs, and medical staffs of the hospitals in the diocese of Richmond as well as the clergy and laity of the diocese. Members are urged to attend all meetings of the commission, may serve as officers and on the executive committee, and may vote on all issues. Associate members shall be appointed annually by the bishop for a term of one year and may serve successive terms. Associate members shall be drawn from the clergy and laity and shall be selected for their expertise or interest in some facet of medical ethics. Associate members will be urged to attend only those meetings of the commission at which their area of expertise or interest will be discussed and for the purposes of counseling the commission members. Associate members shall not hold an office or serve on the executive committee but may vote on issues in their particular area of expertise or interest.

In the event of the resignation of a member or associate member, the bishop may appoint a substitute member or associate member to fill the unexpired term. Furthermore, the bishop may request the resignation of a member or associate member whose conduct is contrary to the objectives of the commission.

Article III
Activities and Functions

The medical ethics commission shall do the following:

1. Be an official diocesan commission reporting on medical-moral issues directly to the bishop; the bishop will relate directly to the hospitals in the diocese

2. Endeavor to create moral leadership in sensitive medical-moral areas in accordance with the *Ethical and Religious Directives for Catholic Health Facilities*

3. Make recommendations to the bishop on the establishment of guidelines for medical ethics committees in each of the diocesan hospitals or health institutions

4. Meet regularly to carry out the above in accordance with the bylaws of the medical ethics commission

Article IV
Meetings

Meetings of the medical ethics commission and the executive committee of the commission shall be held in accordance with the bylaws of the commission.

Article V
Bylaws and Amendments to the Constitution

The bylaws of the medical ethics commission shall be admitted and taken to be its laws subject to the constitution. The bylaws may be amended at any meeting of the Commission by two thirds (2/3) vote of the voting members present or by proxy, provided that a copy of the resolution to amend the bylaws is mailed to each member at least ten (10) days before the meeting, at which such amendment is to be submitted for vote. The constitution may be amended at any meeting of the commission by a two thirds (2/3) vote of the voting members present or by proxy, provided that a copy of the resolution to amend the constitution is mailed to each member at least ten (10) days before the meeting at which such amendment is to be submitted for vote.

Article VI
Liquidation

In the event of the liquidation of the medical ethics commission by the bishop, all funds and records shall be forwarded to the chancery office and will become the property of the diocese of Richmond.

Bylaws
of the
Medical Ethics Commission
Diocese of Richmond

Article I
Commission Year

The operating of the commission shall be from May 1 to April 30.

Article II
Meetings

Regular meetings of the commission shall be held at least four (4) times in each commission year at such time and place as designated by its members. The annual meeting shall be the last of the regular meetings in the commission year. A special meeting may be called at any time by order of the executive committee, and the agenda of the meeting shall be restricted only to that issue(s) for which the meeting is called. Meetings of the executive committee may be called at any time by order of the chairman. At least ten (10) days' notice shall be given by the secretary of the regular and annual meetings At least two (2) days' notice shall be given by the secretary of a special meeting. No notice is required for an executive committee meeting.

Five (5) voting members shall constitute a quorum at regular, annual, and special meetings, provided that at least two (2) of the five (5) voting members are from the administrative staffs of at least two (2) of the diocesan hospitals. A majority of the votes cast by the voting members present or by proxy shall be decisive of any motion or resolution presented, except for the removal of an officer, which would require a two thirds (2/3) vote of the members present or by proxy. Members may vote on all motions, resolutions, and issues in all regular, annual, or special meetings in person or by proxy. Associate members may vote on only those motions, resolutions, and issues relating to their particular area of expertise or interest and only in person.

Article III
Officers and Duties

The officers of the medical ethics commission shall be the chairman, vice chairman, secretary, and treasurer. These officers shall be elected by a plurality vote of the voting members present or by proxy of the annual meeting. They shall take office at the end of the annual meeting and shall serve for 1 year or until their respective successors take office. In the event of a vacancy, the members may elect by plurality vote a substitute officer to fill the unexpired term. Officers shall be eligible for reelection for no more than one (1) successive term. The officers shall constitute the membership of the executive committee. An officer may be removed from office by a two thirds (2/3) vote of the voting members present or by proxy at a regular, annual, or special meeting of the commission. Also, termination of membership will automatically terminate the individual's tenure in office.

The chairman shall be the chief elected officer of the commission and shall preside at all meetings of the commission. It shall be his duty to exercise supervision over the affairs of the commission and to report to the bishop on such affairs. The vice chairman, in the absence of the chairman, shall perform the duties of the latter. The vice chairman may also be assigned duties by the chairman that will allow the vice chairman to become familiar with the duties of the chairman. The secretary shall keep the minutes of all the meetings of the commission, shall notify members and appropriate associate members of meetings, shall maintain a roster of all members and associate members, and shall keep a record of all correspondence and other information relative to the commission. The treasurer shall maintain the funds of the commission and shall report fund transactions to the members at the regular and annual meetings of the commission.

Article IV
Committees

The executive committee shall consist of the chairman, vice chairman, secretary, and treasurer. The executive committee will carry out the affairs of the full commission to the extent that it may not approve motions or resolutions concerning medical-moral issues for implementation in the diocesan hospitals. The nominating committee shall be appointed annually from the members by the chairman before the annual meeting. The committee will select a slate of officers for recommendation to the commission at the annual meeting. Other committees shall be appointed from the members and associate members by the chairman. The purpose of the committees shall be stated at the time of appointment, and the committee shall terminate upon completion of its assigned objectives.

Article V
Dues

In order to carry out the activities of the medical ethics commission, the members shall establish by a plurality vote a reasonable assessment of each diocesan hospital.

Models of Multi-institutional System Committees

| Sample |

System Model 1

Health Care System Corporate Ethics Committee

Purpose

The corporate medical-moral committee is the body responsible for developing and monitoring guidelines to be followed within the member institutions. The local committee of each facility is entrusted with the task of developing and implementing an institutional program of ethics that conforms to the guidelines developed by the corporate committee. The corporate committee is the prime reference group for the corporate ethicist. Although the major focus of this committee is medical-moral, it may also address social justice issues.

Responsibilities

- Assist, advise, and give direction to the corporate ethicist; although the ethicist is not directly accountable to this committee, the committee is a resource and directional board for the ethicist

- Establish and refer to the CEO of the system the medical-moral policy to be implemented in the member institutions regarding medical-moral committees, polices, and procedures

- Raise issues and questions for discussion and determine how the institutional medical-moral committees will address these issues

- Receive and review quarterly reports on institutional medical-moral committees

- Receive questions and issues from the institutional ethicist, the medical-moral committee, and the adminstrator

- Implement a system that provides for annual review of institutional policies

- Convene twice a year the ethicists, chairpersons of ethics committees, and the CEO of each institution

- Invite on a rotating basis institutional ethicists or other consultants to attend the committee meetings at the corporate level

Operational Guidelines

- Meet monthly

- Maintain minutes of all meetings and forward appropriate communications to the CEOs of each facility and to sponsor

Membership

- Two representatives of sponsoring group

- Two corporate officers

- One moral theologian

- One corporate ethicist

- One physician

- One nurse

- One lawyer

- One administrator

In addition, two invitational, rotational members (one institutional ethicist and another expert on a particular subject or topic of discussion) may attend each session but will not have a vote.

Sample

System Model 2
Health Care System Interinstitutional Ethics Committee

Purpose

The purpose of the health care system Interinstitutional ethics committee is to provide a forum for the sharing of educational and policy needs in the areas of ethics as they are experienced by the institutions within the system. The committee is advisory to the corporate staff and does not diminish the right of the local boards to develop policy consistent with Church teaching and the directives of the diocesan bishop.

Functions

- Identify critical medical-moral and social justice issues that may create challenge or difficulty for the institutions

- Share policies and procedures used in the various institutions to address medical-moral issues

- Advise corporate vice president of educational needs experienced at the local level so that he or she may assist in developing the appropriate educational responses

- Advise CEOs of system on those issues that require a position by the system and support corporate staff to both develop and implement such policies

- Review corporate policies and make recommendations about proposed or actual policies to the governing board of the system; these reviews may be requested by a member of the governing board or by institutional CEOs

- Determine what educational programs should be conducted at corporate rather than at institutional level

Membership

The interinstitutional ethics committee shall be composed of the following persons:

- System president

- System vice president of values

- System medical director

- Two representatives of the sponsoring group

- CEO of each institution within system

- One physician from each institution within system

- Institutional ethicist or theologian advisor for each institution

The bishop of each diocese in which a system institution is located is invited to be an honorary member of the committee.

Operational Guidelines

- The committee shall be convened twice a year for two days. The first day shall be concerned with an educational program and the second with communication and sharing among the members.

- Although the committee is advisory, votes will be taken on all issues that are discussed so that the corporate staff understand institutional positions.

- Minutes of all meetings will be kept and copies will be forwarded to corporate officers and the CEO and chairman of the board of each institution.

- The vice president of values will convene and coordinate all committee activities.

Job Descriptions

Job Description

Director of Ethics, Institution

The director of ethics is appointed by the CEO and is accountable to the vice president for mission and philosophy for the coordination of policy education in medical-moral and social ethics issues.

Specific Responsibilities

- To develop and present to all new employees and physicians a statement on the ethical posture of the institution and the implications of that posture on care and service within the institution

- To assess employee needs in areas of ethical education and develop the appropriate programs

- To develop and present to all new employees and physicians a statement on the ethical posture of the institution and the implications of that posture on care and service within the institution

- To assess employee needs in areas of ethical education and

- To maintain "awareness program" so that vital ethical issues are brought before employees, patients, and community on regular basis through a variety of methods

- To develop special ethical education programs for the management team and for the board of trustees at least twice a year

- To attend and participate in medical staff meetings and collaborate with medical director in developing programs for physicians

- To collaborate with other staff in presenting interdisciplinary programs in ethics

- To provide individual consultation to staff, patients, and families as requested or directed by the appropriate administrative officer

- To develop and publicize the "ethical referal system," which allows employees to refer issues to the ethics committees

- To serve as staff to the ethics committee and to have ex-officio membership on the committee

- To coordinate "ethical rounds" conducted on monthly basis

- To represent the institution on the diocesan and system ethics committees

- To initiate ongoing review of existing policies and procedures to ensure that all are consistent with institutional values and philosophy

| Sample |

Job Description

Director of Medical-Moral Affairs, Diocese

The diocese director of medical-moral affairs is appointed by and is directly accountable to the bishop for the coordination of policy and education on medical-moral issues within the diocese.

Specific Responsibilites

- To consult with the bishop on medical-moral issues in general and institutional practice in particular

- To serve as the bishop's representative to the health care facilities within the diocese in medical-moral issues

- To assist in developing and communicating ethical guidelines approved by the bishop for the health care facilities

- To develop diocesan-wide programs in ethics for health care personnel (particularly physicians and nurses) in collaboration with representatives of the health care facilities

- To coordinate educational programs in medical-moral issues for the priests, religious, and laity of diocese

- To convene annually the CEO and the ethicists and the sponsors of each facility in the diocese

- To assist in establishing networking between facilities so that experience may be shared

- To prepare analyses of medical-moral cases submitted to the bishop for review and action

- To monitor legislation at the state and local levels so that appropriate and timely responses can be developed

- To coordinate the activities of the diocesan Christian medical ethics committee

- To meet with institutional adminstrators on a regular basis to ensure effective two-way communication between the diocese and the health care facilities

- To submit to bishop, on a quarterly basis, a report of major issues and activities

| Sample |

Job Description

Director of Ethics, Sponsoring Congregation

The congregation director of ethics is appointed by the major superior and is directly accountable to the major superior or the designated council member. The director is responsible for ensuring that the values of the Church and the congregation are transmitted to and lived out at the system and institutional level; the director is also available to the congregation for educational and consultative services and serves as a consultant to both the congregation and the facilities.

Specific Responsibilities

- To articulate and communicate the congregation's ethical values and stance

- To advise and consult congregational leadership on social justice and medical-moral issues (e.g., clinical practice, investment policies, employee relations)

- To recommend educational programs for the congregation, system or institutional level

- To advise system and institutional personnel on specific ethical issues and assist them in developing corporate policy

- To develop and implement educational programs for the boards of the system and institution

- To consult (when requested by authorized personnel) with physicians, patients, or staff of system or institution

- To anticipate issues, develop responses, and recommend policy to sponsoring group so that corporate stance is determined before a crisis occurs

- To maintain effective communication with ethics personnel at the system, institutional, and diocesan levels

- To provide consultation services to ethics committees at the system and institutional level

- To provide to congregation on an ongoing basis a brief summary and analysis of pressing ethical issues

- To provide to sponsoring congregation on a quarterly basis a report of the ethical situation in each sponsored facility

- To develop and implement on an annual basis a mechanism for evaluating system and institution adherence to the congregation's ethical values

Sample

Job Description

Director of Ethics, Multi-institutional System

The multi-institutional system director of ethics is appointed by and is responsible to the vice president for mission effectiveness (mission services, religious values, Christian effectiveness, or sponsorship activities) and is responsible for education in and implementation of ethical values consistent with the mission of the sponsoring body and the Catholic Church. In addition to medical-moral issues, the director is concerned with general ethical issues of social justice.

Specific Responsibilites

- To maintain the corporate ethics offices with the appropriate tools and resources (reference library, communication vehicles, timelines for program implementation, evaluation mechanism, and so forth)

- To develop and implement a communication system between the corporate office and the ethics personnel at the institutional level

- To review institutional policies and procedures and make recommendations consistent with corporate accountability and institutional autonomy

- To coordinate activities of the corporate ethics committee and ensure appropriate interdisciplinary and institutional representation

- To develop educational program in ethics for corporate board and staff and for institutional boards and personnel as requested

- To assist in the formation and development of ethics committees within the health care facilities

- To convene chairpersons of institutional ethics committees at least twice a year

- To maintain a listing of appropriate resources for various ethical issues
- To assist in recruiting and evaluating institutional ethicists or consultants

- To develop and recommend systemwide policies for consideration by the corporate board

- To prepare for corporate staff quarterly summaries of major ethical issues and activities experienced at system and institutional level

- To establish networks with Catholic conference representatives and health associations of states in which facilities are located so that issues will be identified and responded to appropriately and in a timely fashion

- To serve as consultant to sponsor, corporate board, or institutional executives when requested

Glossary for Ethics Committees

Bioethical. Signifies ethical considerations in topics related to biology, e.g., in medicine or health care.

Conscience. Faculty that distinguishes right and wrong in one's conduct.

Ethical and Religious Directives for Catholic Health Facilities. Guidelines and rules approved in November 1971 and revised by the National Conference of Catholic Bishops (NCCB) to ensure spiritual service and medical practice in accord with Catholic Church teaching.

Ethically ordinary means of prolonging life. All medicines, treatments, and operations that offer the patient a reasonable hope of benefit and can be obtained and used without excessive expense, pain, or other burden.

Ethically extraordinary means of prolonging life. All medicines, treatments, and operations that cannot be obtained or used without excessive expense, pain, or other burden for the patient or others, or which would not offer the patient a reasonable hope of benefit.

Ethicist. An expert in the knowledge and application of ethics.

Christian ethicist (also called moral theologian). An expert in the knowledge and application of Christian ethics.

Ethics (also called moral philosophy). Study of human behavior with reference to standards of right and wrong, including specific moral choices an individual makes in dealing with others.

Christian ethics (also called moral theology). Study of ethics that includes Christian revelation as a source of knowledge and principles about the human person, human behavior, and human relationships.

Ethics committee functions. Activities of ethics committees. In Catholic health facilities these are primarily recommending policy, providing ethical education for staff, consulting and making decisions on specific ethical issues and cases.

Exceptionless moral norms. Norms for human behavior that are so basic to the meaning and purpose of human existence and human interrelations that they identify the inherent moral character of specific human actions which cannot be altered by particular circumstances or motives (e.g., direct abortion is always wrong).

Institutional conscience. An institution's articulation of right and wrong behavior through the ethical principles its leaders adopt.

Institutional review board (IRB). Institutional committees mandated by federal regulation for all institutions receiving federal funds for research on human subjects. Their major objective is to ensure informed consent and positive risk-benefit ratio. Such committees to oversee the medical care of infants have also been proposed in response to the Doe cases.

Liability. An institution's or individual's responsibility for actions and omissions, including those of subordinates and employees.

Magisterium. The competence of the Catholic Church, exercised by the pope and bishops in union with him, to teach in matters of faith and morals with the authority of Christ.

Medical-moral committees. Committees in health care facilities that review questions of medical ethics.

Moral rights and responsibilities. Rights and responsibilities that belong to human persons because of their unique, inherent dignity and potential.

National Conference of Catholic Bishops (NCCB). Assembly of the Church hierarchy of the United States and its territories; its purpose is to foster bishops' collegial concern for the Church and society in the United States and throughout the world.

Sacred Congregation for the Doctrine of the Faith. A teaching commission of the Catholic Church under the pope's direct supervision. Its purpose is to respond to doctrinal and moral questions by clarifying Catholic teaching.

Social justice. The equitable distribution of goods and the recognition of the rights so that each individual has the opportunity to fulfill his or her human dignity and contribute to the common good.

Bibliography

Allen, P.A., et al. "Development of An Ethical Committee and Effects on a Research Design," *Lancet*, 1(May 29, 1982): 1233-1236.

Bader, Sr. D., OP., "Medical-Moral Committees: Guarding Values in an Ambivalent Society," *Hospital Progress*, 63(Dec. 1982): 80-83.

Breur, H. et al. "Role of Ethical Guidance Committees in Clinical Research," *Controlled Clinical Trials*, (May 1981): 421-427.

Campbell, J.D., et al. "The Hospital Ethics Committee," *Medical Journal of Australia*, 1(Feb. 21, 1980): 168-169.

Cebik, L.B. "The Professional Role and Clinical Education of the Medical Ethicist," *Ethics, Science, and Medicine*, 6(1979). 115-121.

Cohen, C.B. "Interdisciplinary Consultation on the Care of the Critically Ill and Dying: The Role of One Hospital's Ethics Committee," *Critical Care Medicine*, 10(Nov. 1982): 776-784.

Cranford, Ronald and E. Edward Doudera. "The Emergence of Institutional Ethics Committees," *Law, Medicine, and Health Care* 12(Feb. 1984): 13-20.

Denham, M.J. et al. "Work of a District Ethical Committee," *British Medical Journal*, 2(Oct. 27, 1979): 1042-1045.

Esqueda, K. "Hospital Ethics Committees: Four Case Studies," *Hospital Medical Staff*, 7(Nov. 1978): 26-30.

Fleischman, A. and T. Murray. "Ethics Committee for Infants Doe?" *Hastings Center Report*, (Dec. 1983): 5-9.

Freedman, B. "One Philosopher's Experience on an Ethics Committee," *Hastings Center Report*, 11(Apr. 1981): 20-22.

Glaser, J., ed. "A Model for Forming a Medical-Moral Committee," *Ethic Notes*, Farmington, MI: Sisters of Mercy Health Corp., 1981.

"Guidelines to Aid Ethical Committees Considering Research in Children: Working Party on Ethics of Research in Children," *British Medical Journal*, 280(Jan. 1980): 229-236.

"Guidelines to Ethical Committees Considering Research Involving Children," *Archives of Diseases in Childhood*, 55(Jan. 1980): 75-77.

Guidi, D.J., ed. *Hospital Ethics Committees: Potential Mediators for Educational and Policy Change*, Dissertation, Fairleigh Dickinson University, 1983. 201 pp.

Hamilton, M.P. "Role of an Ethicist in the Conduct of Clinical Trials in the U.S.," *Controlled Clinical Trials*, (May 1981): 411-420.

Hirsch, H. "Establish Ethics Committees to Minimize Liability, Authority Advises," *Hospital Risk Management*, 3(Apr. 1981): 45-48.

Holmes, C. "Bioethical Decision-Making An Approach to Improve the Process," *Medical Care* 17(Nov. 1979): 1131-1138.

John Paul II, Pope. "A Patient is a Person," *Medical Services*, 39(Feb. 1982): 13-17 passim.

Kalchbrenner, Sr. J., et al. "Ethics Committees and Ethicists in Catholic Hospitals," *Hospital Progress* 64(Sept. 1983): 77-81.

Keenan, C. "Ethics Committees: Trend for Troubling Times," *The Hospital Medical Staff*, 12(June 1983): 2-11.

Knight, E. and J. Moore. *To Be or Not To Be Involved: The Role of Hospital Trustees and Management in Bio-Ethical Decision Making*, Edmonton: Alberta Hospital Association, 1983.

Levine, C. "Hospital Ethics Committee a Guarded Prognosis," *Hastings Center Report* 7(June 1977): 25-26.

Levine, M.D., et al. "Ethical Rounds in a Children's Medical Center: Evaluation of a Hospital Based Program for Continued Education in Medical Ethics," *Pediatrics*, 60(Aug. 1977): 253-255.

Lisson, Edward, SJ. "Active Medical Morals Committee: Valuable Resources for Health Care," *Hospital Progress*, 63(Oct. 1982): 36-37, 68.

Lo. B., et al. "Frequency of Ethical Dilemmas in Medical In-Patient Service," *Archives of Internal Medicine*, 141(July 1981): 1062-1064.

Lobo, G. "Medical Ethics Forum," *Medical Services*, 36(Nov.-Dec. 1977): 37, 39.

_____. "Medical Ethics Forum-22 Models for Christian Hospitals," *Medical Service*, 38(Nov.-Dec. 1981): 23, 27-28, 31.

MacIntyre, A. "Theology, Ethics, and the Ethics of Medicine and Health Care: Comments on Papers by Novak, Mouw, Roach, Cahill, and Hart," *Journal of Medicine and Philosophy*, (Dec. 1979): 435-443.

Mazonson, P.D., et al. "Medical Ethical Rounds: Development and Organization," *Rocky Mountain Medical Journal*, 76(Nov.-Dec. 1979): 282-288.

"Medical Societies Propose Life Preservation Committees: Maryland," *Hospitals*, 49(Aug. 16, 1975): 227.

Murphy, M.A. and J. Murphy. "Making Ethical Decisions Systematically," *Nursing* '76. 6(May 1976): 13.

O'Rourke, K., OP. "Ethical Committees in Hospitals," *Ethical Issues in Health Care, St. Louis University Medical Center*, (Aug. 1983).

Pinkus, R.L. "Medical Foundations of Various Approaches to Medical-Ethic Decision-Making," *Journal of Medicine and Philosophy*, 6(Aug. 1981): 295-307.

Pope John XXIII Medical-Moral Research and Education Center. "How Can Medical-Moral Committees Function Effectively in Catholic Health Facilities?" *Hospital Progress*, 64(Apr. 1983): 77-78.

President's Commission for the Study of Ethical Problems in Medicine and Biomedical and Behavioral Research. *Deciding to Forego Life-Sustaining Treatment*, Washington DC: Government Printing Office, 1983, Appendix F: 440-457.

Randal, J. "Are Ethics Committees Alive and Well?" *Hastings Center Report*, (Dec. 1983): 10-12.

Somfai, B. "Moral Leadership in a Socialized Health Care System," (Part II) *CHAC Review*, 8(Jan.-Feb. 1980): 24-26.

Stalder, G. "Ethical Committees in a Pediatric Hospital," *European Journal of Pediatrics*, 136(May 1981): 119-122.

Teel, K. "The Physician's Dilemma, A Doctor's View: What the Law Should Be," *Baylor Law Review* 27(Winter 1975): 6-9.

Veatch, R.M. "What is the Scope of Hospital Ethics Committees?" *Hospital Medical Staff*, (Summer 1977): 24-30.

_____. "Hospital Ethics Committees: Is There A Role?" *Hastings Center Report*, (June 1977): 22, 25.

Wallace, C. "Outcry over Baby Doe may reverse little used hospital ethics' committees," *Modern Healthcare*, 13(Sept. 1983): 78, 80.

Weisman, S.A. "Nursing Home Experience with an Ethics Committee," *Nursing Homes*, 29(Sept.-Oct. 1980): 2-4.

Younger, S., et al. "Patients' Attitudes Toward Hospital Ethics Committees," *Law, Medicine, and Health Care*, 12(Feb. 1984): 21-25.